To Dav[...]
Fellow



The Schizoid World of Jean-Paul Sartre and R.D. Laing

Warmest wishes
Douglas
Nov. 06

# The Schizoid World of Jean-Paul Sartre and R.D. Laing

Douglas Kirsner

KARNAC
New York
London

First softcover printing 2003

10 9 8 7 6 5 4 3 2 1

Published by Karnac USA, an imprint of Other Press LLC.  Printed in the United States of America on acid-free paper. For information write to Other Press LLC, 307 Seventh Avenue, Suite 1807, New York, NY 10001. Or visit our website: www.otherpress.com.

Library of Congress Cataloging-in-Publication Data

Kirsner, Douglas.
The schizoid world of Jean-Paul Sartre and R.D. Laing / Douglas Kirsner.
p. cm.
Originally published: St. Lucia, Qld. : University of Queensland Press, 1976.
Includes bibliographical references and index.
ISBN 1-59051-051-8 (pbk.)
1. Sartre, Jean-Paul, 1905- 2. Laing, R. D. (Ronald David), 1927- I. Title.

B2430.S34 K45 2003
194—dc21

2002032171

# Contents

# Acknowledgments

I should like to thank Alastair Davidson, Max Charlesworth, Alan Davies, Diane Wieneke and Maurita Harney for the assistance they have given me with this work. I am grateful for the encouragement that the late Ron Jackson gave me. I want, also, to express my gratitude to my parents for their very valuable help.

D.K.

*He could have resigned himself to a prison. To end as a prisoner—that could be a life's ambition. But it was a barred cage that he was in. Calmly and insolently, as if at home, the din of the world streamed out and in through the bars, the prisoner was really free, he could take part in everything, nothing that went on outside escaped him, he could simply have left the cage, the bars were yards apart, he was not even a prisoner.*

Franz Kafka

# Introduction

At seventy Sartre is nearly blind and has been forced by circumstance to abandon his life's work as a writer. His work on Flaubert which aimed at reaching the lived experience of that writer, situating him both in terms of his time and his personal history and projects, remains unfinished although the essentials are done. But, as Sartre points out, the work of all writers remains incomplete. In fact the very nature of human existence means our contingency, our mortality which stand in the face of our thirst for the absolute. Sartre, who had prophesied that he would end his life as he had begun it: among books, is now victim to this facticity. His work as a writer is over, he accepts it and feels that he has said what he has had to say. He continues to work on dialogues and politics and hopes to have another ten effective years ahead of him. However the basic framework of this remarkable writer, philosopher and political activist who has been among the foremost intellectuals of our time, is complete.[1]

In this book I want to develop an immanent critique of this framework attempting to situate Sartre and his work in relation to his epoch and biography in a way which itself presents some parallels with the methods Sartre himself proposed in *Search for a Method* and used in his work on Flaubert. Sartre will be seen as a man of his time and also in his specificity, as having travelled a certain path which can be understood as constituting itself as a unity. Sartre at seventy remains true to the basic concerns and principles of his early

1. *See* Michel Contat's extensive interviews with Sartre (1975), partially published in *Le Nouvel Observateur*. Abridged versions of these interviews also appear in the London *Observer* and in *The New York Review of Books*. The interviews appear in full in Sartre, *Situations* X, Gallimard, Paris 1976. (For volume numbers, dates and publishing details of this and subsequent footnotes, *see* bibliography.)

life, although these are of course very much further developed. His work may be seen as constantly spiralling through the same nodal points although doing so at different levels. He has constantly maintained that man is freedom and, if a label were to be applied to him, he would today still prefer to be called "existentialist" rather than "Marxist". Sartre does not like to be labelled, to be institutionalized or for others to have power over him. This is in line with the anarchism which he admits has consistently informed his life's work. But he is profoundly aware of the influence of circumstances in shaping the individual subject. Asked in a recent interview how he would like to be remembered, he replies with the names of works ranging from *Nausea* to *The Critique of Dialectical Reason* and adds:

> As a man if a certain Jean-Paul Sartre is remembered, I would like people to remember the milieu or historical situation in which I lived, the general characteristics of this milieu, how I lived in it, in terms of all the aspirations which I tried to gather up within myself.[2]

Laing too has traversed a definite path, though it has taken a curious twist of late. He now practices psychotherapy in London after having journeyed from psychiatry to mysticism, culminating in a lengthy meditative stay in a Buddhist monastery in Ceylon from which he returned in late 1972. The reader of his last writings before his stay in Ceylon could be surprised by Laing's subsequent modification of his mysticism. Indeed Laing today traces psychotherapy back to "the very roots of western medicine and it is in the fundamental tradition of Aesculapian medicine".[3] This comes from a man who had previously seen the illness model as extremely socially oppressive. His later works had progressively discarded the medical-psychiatric—even existential psychological—view of mental illness. So much was this so that the schizophrenic could be seen as a prophet and seer and the psychiatrist as someone institutionalizing society's invalidation and suppression of people's true other selves. In a way Laing seems latterly to have turned back to some of the conceptions of *The Divided Self*. It is quite possible to view his work and its development in terms of the work which led up to the

2. Max Charlesworth, *The Existentialists and Jean-Paul Sartre*, p.154. This book contains a number of original interviews including ones with Sartre and Laing. It serves moreover as a valuable introduction to existentialism and its background. Also useful in this context is R.C. Solomon, *From Rationalism to Existentialism: The Existentialists and Their Nineteenth Century Background*. Edgar Friedenberg's *Laing*, is a small book which may prove a useful introduction to Laing.
3. Charlesworth, ibid., p.52.

journey to Ceylon, and to see in it an underlying framework. Since his return there is no reason to suspect any radical departure from some of his previous positions and outlooks: that is, his post-Ceylon attitudes can be seen in terms of his pre-Ceylon views. Moreover in contrast with Sartre for whom there is a large mass of biographical and autobiographical material, there is a noticeable lack of personal information about Laing. I think that his belief-systems and the about-face after his stay in Ceylon could be explicable in terms of Laing's own emotional development at least on one level. Laing has written two books since his return from Ceylon, both of which are being published by Penguin Books in 1976. Entitled *Why Did the Peacock Scream*? and *The Facts of Life: an Essay in Feelings, Facts and Fantasies*, they constitute refreshing attempts to reach lived reality outside the confines of disciplinary boundaries. Originally *The Facts of Life* bore the subtitle of *An Essay in Existential Biology* which Laing later changed because he thought it too pretentious. Nevertheless this subtitle well illustrates his current concerns which are to give an account of human experience that does justice both to experiential reality and biological fact. This is not far removed from the interest of *The Divided Self* although Laing has lately attempted to trace childhood experience back to its pre-natal interuterine origins. But this existential psychiatrist is not the seer of *The Politics of Experience* nor the Eastern mystic of *Knots*. Laing is chairman of the Philadelphia Association which has a number of functioning communities, trains existential therapists and runs seminars in phenomenology. His post-Ceylon views constitute quite a contrast with his immediately previous work and is more in tune with the themes of his earlier work. In this book I shall describe Laing's journey—which I take as encapsulating the schizoid plight of millions—in terms basically of his published clinical and intellectual research. His work will be seen as itself developing within the schizoid framework it depicts.

Sartre and Laing confront many of the same sorts of problems and deal with them from similar standpoints. According to Laing, Sartre had been writing out of the same tradition that he had been immersed in, and was a

> big vessel afloat in the same ocean that I was trying to keep afloat in myself ... It was through Sartre that I was impelled to get hold of Husserl and Hegel. Sartre's earlier work was newer to me and perhaps in a way more formative in the sense that it was a gate-opener to the tradition that Sartre espoused, Hegel, Husserl and Heidegger.[4]

4. Ibid., p.49.

Laing regards Sartre's later work in particular as providing as decisive a framework for demystification of the human condition as Freud and Marx had constructed in their day.[5] He found Sartre's theoretical concepts there "extremely useful" in his study of families.[6] Much of Laing's work is suffused with Sartrean terminology and concepts. It addresses itself as much to the micro-systems of dyadic and family relations as it does to the problems of individual identity and ontological security in the world that Sartre describes so compellingly as being systematically outside our collective control.

Sartre for his part admires the work of Laing in locating "mental illness" within Sartrean social categories and is completely in favour of Laing's anti-psychiatry.[7] But it would be mistaken to view Laing as having simply developed and applied certain Sartrean categories. For while both Sartre and Laing agree on the landscape of *The Critique of Dialectical Reason*, Sartre is no mystic and Laing no radical political activist. Their problematics are similar, their solutions are not.

Both Sartre and Laing are concerned with the way the individual relates with the social systems he lives, especially those systems that constitute mediations between the individual and the social totality. These extend synchronically through a hierarchy of interrelating contextual systems of family through class to culture, and historically through the past relations of the individual, especially with his family in his early years. The locus of these concerns is the biography of the person using Sartre's progressive-regressive method in comprehending how the individual shapes his life in a world which shapes him. But neither Sartre nor Laing wants to dispense with individual subjectivity, regarding it as essential to a human study of human beings. They both wish to salvage this subjectivity throughout their work: even for the latest Sartre "freedom is the very definition of man",[8] and for Laing the individual never need cease searching for transcendence. Indeed they both share a conception of what it is to be truly a self.

Sartre is firmly embedded in the Cartesian tradition of French intellectual culture which takes the reality of the *cogito* as its foundation. This is exemplified in Valery's desire to reach *le moi pur* voided of passions and adventitious ideas. Sartre's interest in extreme situations showing me who I really am, his concern over the

5. R.D. Laing and D.G. Cooper (1964), *Reason and Violence: A Decade of Sartre's Philosophy*, p.10.
6. Charlesworth, *The Existentialists*, p.47.
7. Ibid., pp.127-28.
8. Ibid., p.25.

inevitable intrusion of the other into my inner world and with the near impossibility of authentic relationships of reciprocity between people are all symptomatic of his view of subjectivity as inviolable core. The self is what I am when the other is totally excluded—the extent to which I am constituted by others is that to which I am not myself. Total aloneness and fusion are the two exhaustive alternatives for Sartre, rather than being the two extremes of a continuum along which most relationships may be situated. For Sartre relationships necessarily involve theft: the real self for Sartre is alone. His love-hate relationship with Freud is founded on Sartre's fascination with Freud's explanations of individual behaviour, together with his horror at the realization that consciousness may not be in control (although it is not in control either in his own philosophy which might be seen as substituting the domination of the other for that of the id.)

Laing's view of the self devolves around the same issues. The self is impinged upon so far, Laing asserts in his later work, that the salvation of the true self can come only through the transformation of the ordinary self into another. The true/false self dichotomy, inherited from Winnicott, is used by Laing to connote an alienation so radical that the emergence of the true self is dependent on mystical experience, not on psychoanalytical therapy. It may be noted that Laing like Sartre uses isolation and fusion as the only real possibilities for human life today. However self-fulfilment lies in losing oneself in a transcendental voyage which may be interpreted in terms of merging with the good mother once again after having suffered the pain of being cut off from her in a hostile world.

While Sartre and Laing share a concern for rescuing subjectivity in a dehumanized world, and about the possibility of reciprocal relationships in a bad social whole, their basic premises about the nature of this subjectivity may well be called into question. The person has been split into mind and body, and the mind then stripped of its social accretions in a search for a true self. The conceptions of self postulated by Sartre and Laing serve as last-ditch stands against an otherwise seemingly overwhelming and hostile world, though I see the genesis of these very conceptions as distortion of human reality through the defences of splitting, denial and idealization of what it is to be a self. I contend that the basic framework that exists from individual through to macro-social systems is a schizoid one—that there is a failure of basic trust in the self and in the general social contexts as being sufficiently good and reliable for authentic autonomy and mature relationship to develop. When schizoid phenomena are understood contextually, they may be seen as systemic manifestations of a deeply rooted and widespread, self-inflicted malaise of the human context itself.

The search for identity and ontological security indicate the problem of their very scarcity in contemporary life, and if the problems Sartre and Laing depict represent false ways of seeing, they are certainly widespread ones. Moreover it is not sufficient to dispel illusions, but to understand them as produced by men and as involving the need to transform the conditions requiring such illusions.[9] Sartre and Laing may be seen as expressing many of the problems of our time, as supplying many profound insights while at the same time exhibiting the ramifications of these very problems. Sartre and Laing's thirst for the absolute together with the disillusionment with the death of God may be seen as conditioned by the experience of this radically alienated world in which the individual seems to have no room, and which is not experienced as good enough to sustain him properly.

How is it possible to understand an individual writer both in his particularity and as an expression of his time? How is it possible to integrate the psychological with the sociological without doing injustice to either by reductionism? These are questions with which Laing and particularly Sartre grapple.

In *Search for a Method* Sartre introduces the vital concept of mediation which helps account for the individual biography systemically without making him a mere reflex of his time. Biography may be seen as situated between psychology and sociology: "Valery is a petit-bourgeois intellectual, no doubt about it. But not every petit-bourgeois intellectual is Valery".[10] The importance of childhood and of individual projects within larger social contexts has been neglected by traditional Marxists and conventional sociologists, according to Sartre.

Cross-reference of mediating contexts is provided for in Sartre's "progressive-regressive method" which aims at progressively determining the biography of the individual in terms of his aims and regressing to an understanding of the circumstances and background in which these projects are undertaken: it determines the biography by studying the period and the period through the individual biography. If we regress to understanding the childhood of Flaubert, for exam-

9. *See* Karl Marx, "Towards a Critique of Hegel's Philosophy of Law: Introduction" in L.D. Easton and K.H. Guddat (eds.), *Writings of the Young Marx on Philosophy and Society*, p.250.
10. J-P. Sartre (1960), *Search for a Method (Question de méthode)*, p.56.

ple, and systematically cross-reference it with what we know of the period, we may be able to progressively reconstruct the situation of the subject who wrote *Madame Bovary*, and reach the depths of lived experience. The original complexity, meaning and richness of past acts is found again. This concept of lived experience (*le vécu*) is used in the work on Flaubert of which Sartre says:

> I would like the reader to feel the presence of Flaubert the whole time; my ideal would be that the reader simultaneously feels, comprehends and knows the personality of Flaubert totally as an individual and yet totally as an expression of his time. In other words, Flaubert can be understood by his difference from his neighbours ... My aim is to try to demonstrate the encounter between the development of the person, as psychoanalysis has shown it to us, and the development of history. For at a certain moment, an individual in his very deepest and most intimate conditioning, by his family, can fulfil a historical role.[11]

Flaubert did not simply react to his time by becoming what was expected of him, but by surpassing his conditioning, as did Genet, in becoming a writer. In the first volume of *The Idiot of the Family* Sartre attempts to deal with the problem of how an individual can be locked in by his neurosis and yet write—a problem which is of course Sartre's own as well. The world Sartre depicts is dark, yet not altogether hopeless, if only because he can write about it. The executive function of this writing will be seen in chapter 3 of this book as standing in contrast with the world portrayed in the writing itself, that is they are split off from each other. Sartre's world is revealed not only in the contents of his writing but in his surpassing them in some ways through his projects as a writer. This effectively means that it is perhaps possible for the individual to escape from the destiny for which he is programmed by the conjuncture of personal and general social neuroses.[12] Individual freedom can never be completely eliminated and constitutes a cornerstone of Sartre's world view, although this freedom can be scarcely in fact exercised and constitutes today "the small movement which makes of a totally conditioned social being someone who does not render back completely what his conditioning has given him".[13]

According to Sartre, everybody agrees that sociology and psychoanalysis should be able to be combined through finding the necessary mediations. "Everybody in fact *says* it, but who has tried to *do*

11. Sartre (1969), "Itinerary of a Thought" (interview), *New Left Review* 58, p.51.
12. Sartre (1972), *L'Idiot de la famille: Gustave Flaubert de 1821 à 1857*.III.
13. Sartre, Itinerary of a Thought, p.145.

it?" Sartre asks, and adds: "The idea of the book on Flaubert was to abandon these theoretical disquisitions, because they were ultimately getting us nowhere, and try to give a concrete example of how it might be done. The result can take care of itself".[14] I entirely agree with Sartre's approach here and I hope the reader will find in this work its own justification.

14. Ibid., p.51.

# PART I

# JEAN-PAUL SARTRE

# 1

# Sisyphean Freedom

Philosophy has long sought an understanding of man and his relationship with the universe; latterday existentialism has subverted the traditional alliance between philosophy and science in favour of one between philosophy and literature.[1] The appropriate "science" for describing human reality cannot be the statistical quantification of the given reality, although this is itself an expression of that reality. The world of literature, however, touches far deeper bases than do statistics—the time is reflected through its literature and through the artists' sensitive response to the prevailing reality. Literature is an expression of what people are—their conflicts and confusions, their hopes and fears, their problems and delights, their goals and values. Literature is a true "science" here in the sense that it deals with knowledge appropriate to its field. If that field is human reality, then the extent to which mechanical precision seems appropriate to the description of human relations now indicates the degree of dehumanization of these relationships.

The novels of Kafka portray the despairing and dehumanized state of modern culture, as do the many works of the existentialist writers. Glicksberg maintains that twentieth century literature is characterized both by Promethean defiance and Sisyphean despair. He observes that this literature illustrates the "central paradox" of the tragic vision of our day: "The suffering that tragedy enacts makes us face the truth in all its terror and grandeur of the human situation, and relies on the moral strength to rise reborn out of the grave of despair."[2]

1. R. Cumming, "The Literature of Extreme Situations" in M. Phillipson (ed.) *Aesthetics Today*, pp. 408-9. (*See* bibliographical note i.e., treatment of footnote material.)
2. C.I. Glicksberg, *The Tragic Vision in Twentieth Century Literature*, p.3.

There seems to be an especially strong need this century for man to make some sense out of his existence. Never has he seen more clearly and felt more powerless. There is a great need for systems to make order out of chaos, and while mass totalitarian ideologies have responded to this need (as well as creating it!), there have also been a large number of philosophies of existence.

In a world in which the time-honoured verities of tradition have been largely superseded and discarded, there has not been a trans-valuation of values, but rather a pervasive feeling of existential anxiety or emptiness, particularly in the most highly "developed" countries.

Dostoevski's phrase, "If God did not exist, everything would be permitted" could not be appropriate in a century where everything has been permitted, the most obvious and extreme forms of totalitarian terror being symptomatic of the almost universal psychological terrorism which leaves the individual with no authentic room to move in his godless world. There has been a variety of responses to this situation. One important and typical interpretation is Camus' version of the myth of Sisyphus. Camus states that the only "truly philosophical problem" is that of suicide.[3] There is no absolute or eternal meaning to life, and the meaning life has is that which we give it. The point that is most important is that our century has been one not only of growing mystification, bureaucratization and implicit and explicit terror, but also one of demystification and growing consciousness. The myth of Sisyphus which depicts Sisyphus eternally pushing a rock to the top of a hill only to let it roll down again, is the image of our existence according to Camus. He writes:

> If this myth is tragic, that is because its hero is conscious. What would his torture be, indeed, if at every step the hope of succeeding upheld him? The workman of today works every day in his life at the same tasks, and this fate is no less absurd. But it is tragic only at the rare moments when it becomes conscious. Sisyphus, proletarian of the gods, powerless and rebellious, knows the whole extent of this wretched condition: it is what he thinks of during his descent. The lucidity that was to constitute his torture at the same time crowns his victory. There is no fate that cannot be surmounted by scorn.[4]

Sisyphus is frighteningly aware of his condition, and it is this awareness which constitutes his suffering. In the past, people had

3. A. Camus, *The Myth of Sisyphus and Other Essays*, p.3.
4. Ibid., pp. 89-90.

believed in ideologies which placed themselves and their activities in a meaningful context. The feelings of "ontological insecurity" are widespread this century in which many people do not know where they are going. Yet it is maintained that the human situation could not be clearer: it has been illuminated, clarified, disclosed, demystified, demythologized, disillusioned, revealed, uncovered. Psychoanalysis and sociology have revealed the depths of our lack of control of our situation, and Freud's hysterical patients have largely been replaced by people suffering various degrees of apathy, unrelatedness, depersonalization, loneliness, derealization, emptiness and existential *angst*.[5] Where God is dead in men's souls, there seems the greater need for a metaphysics which will somehow locate man in a meaningful way. Man's position is elucidated and articulated most clearly when he seems to be most impotent: Scarcely a happy scene.

For Sartre, man is his freedom. Human reality as described by Sartre entirely transcends the traditional disciplinary approaches to it and is itself the basic datum for inquiry. Sartre's work subverts the bases for distinctions among the disciplines through an ultimate understanding of man as freedom. The very emphasis on freedom points to the problems of freedom in this age. There are seemingly overwhelming social forces set in motion which would enslave and determine man. The problem of freedom is uppermost in this century, since it is this freedom that is at stake; the problem of the meaning of this freedom arises in situations in which meaning seems to have disappeared. For Sartre, there is always a gap between the world and myself, and we cannot escape this nothingness which is ourselves. We cannot *be* anything at all, but in the face of immensely powerful forces which would capture, imprison and crush us, our ontological constitution as nothingness is precisely the disaster which we may turn into a triumph.

Sartrean man is a truly Sisyphean figure: he can not only survive but fight despite the gods who wish to dominate him entirely. Extreme or boundary situations show this clearly; we are stripped naked and cannot hide our condition from ourselves as can the "normal" person in "normal" circumstances. What in former times was seen as a caricature or mystification of freedom—that we can be free even in chains—has become for Sartre the testament to our irreducibility. Even under the extreme pressures of the hell and damnation Sartre takes to be contemporary earthly life, men need not be

5. *See* H. Ruitenbeek (ed.) *Psychoanalysis and Existential Philosophy*, Introductory Essay.

compliant victims. There is still an inner core which can refuse to submit and maintain a somewhat demiurgic stoicism. For Sisyphean man may well be obliged to carry out the commands of the gods—the gods may dominate him, but not possess him. Thrown back on his resources, Sisyphean man becomes supremely conscious of his powerlessness against an overwhelming reality; yet in these circumstances where the odds are stacked so surely against him, he can still refuse to be engulfed. Human reality is revealed behind traditional approaches as freedom.

Life is to be understood in the contexts in which it is situated, whether they be termed psychological, sociological or whatever. Sartre puts this dramatically:

> We are not greatly concerned with psychology ... For us psychology is the most abstract of the sciences because it studies the workings of our passions without plunging them back into their true human surroundings, without their background of religious and moral values, the taboos and commandments of society, the conflicts of nations and classes, of rights, of wills, of actions. For us a man is a whole enterprise in himself. And passion is part of that enterprise.[6]

And more succinctly:

> We do not reject psychology, that would be absurd; we integrate life.[7]

Praising Nathalie Sarraute's "anti-novel", Sartre points to Sarraute's technique "which makes it possible to attain, over and beyond the psychological, human reality in its very existence".[8] He believes that "no situation should be analyzed exclusively on the psychological level",[9] and that "it is not a question of instincts or inborn tendencies; what counts is a man's relationship with society, with his family, with everything around him".[10] This is not the preserve of psychology. Sartre says, "I am not at all fond of the word psychological. There is no such thing as the psychological. Let us say that one can improve the biography of the person".[11]

Sartre has written biographies of French writers, seeking an understanding of the setting of their "original choice" of themselves. Baudelaire's "initial choice" of himself was to "exist for himself as he was for others". Once this choice of life project in childhood is es-

6. J.-P. Sartre (1946), "Forgers of Myths: the Young Playwrights of France" *Théâtre Arts*, p. 326.
7. Ibid., p. 329.
8. Sartre (1948), "Nathalie Sarraute" in Sartre, *Situations*, p. 202.
9. Sartre (1961), "Sartre talks to Tynan I", *Observer*.
10. Sartre (1961), "Sartre talks to Tynan II", *Observer*.
11. Sartre (1957), "Interview with Oliver Todd", *Listener*, p. 915.

tablished, thereafter "everything becomes clear".[12] In his mammoth work on Genet, Sartre attempted

> to indicate the limits of psychoanalytical interpretation and Marxist explanation and to demonstrate that freedom alone can account for a person in his totality; to show this freedom at grips with destiny, crushed at first by its mischances, then turning upon them and digesting them little by little; to prove that genius is not a gift but the way out that one invents in desperate cases, to learn the choice that a writer makes of himself of his life, and of the meaning of the universe ... to review in detail the history of his liberation.[13]

Indeed the importance of this freedom is its transcending power:

> We are not lumps of clay; and what is important is not what people make of us, but what we ourselves make of what they have made of us.[14]

Thus the "original choice" is made on the basis of a certain personal and social environment which does not determine but lays the conditions for the range and direction of the life ahead. It is imperative to retrace a life to the decisive choice in childhood and give a "phenomenological description of it".[15] Phenomenological, because "to adopt a mental attitude is to place oneself in a prison without bars".[16] Constricting and confining situations according to preconceived rules and notions can divide, distort and mute a reality which would otherwise cry out to be understood as a unity. Existential phenomenology aims at doing justice to men who are always situated yet free. No matter how alienated he is, a man remains a man.[17]

Man's freedom is revealed to him even—in fact especially—in extreme situations according to Sartre. For example, Orestes knows and proclaims that he is free in the face of the wrath of the gods and the people of Argos. Weighed down by the crime of knowing his freedom, exiled, alone and lonely as a leper, a king without a kingdom, Orestes, zealously followed by the Furies, scorns the gods in pursuit of a new and strange life, which, with patience, would take him well beyond the rivers and mountains towards himself.[18] Orestes in true Sisyphean fashion scorns the gods, where others would give in to them. At the very moment that Orestes sees

12. Sartre (1947), *Baudelaire*, p. 184.
13. Sartre (1952), *Saint Genet: Actor and Martyr*, p. 584.
14. Ibid., p. 49.
15. Ibid., p. 51.
16. Ibid., p. 69.
17. Sartre (1960), *Search for a Method*, pp. 76, 100, 135, 140ff.
18. Sartre (1943), *The Flies*, pp. 312-16.

the strength of the forces against him, he senses his own inner freedom which can never be captured.

*The Flies* was an allegory about the Occupation. The extreme situation of the Occupation could disclose man's essential freedom to him in a way he would not normally see. Sartre wrote:

> Never were we freer than under the German Occupation. We had lost all our rights, and first of all our right to speak ... Everywhere ... we found that filthy and insipid image of ourselves which the oppressor wished to present us. And because of all this, we were free. The more the Nazi venom crept into our thoughts, the more each precise thought was a conquest.[19]

A "republic of silence" was established in which everyone who knew something important to the Resistance asked himself in anguish "If they torture me, can I hold on?". Sartre adds:

> Thus indeed was the question of liberty brought to the very edge of the profoundest comprehension that man can have of himself. For the secret of man is not in his Oedipus or inferiority complex; it is in the power to resist suffering up to the point of death.

He wondered whether the liberation which would bring with it "the republic of the bright day" would "preserve in its sunlight the austere virtues of the republic of silence and the night".[20] This extreme or boundary situation had made self-deception very difficult indeed and had brought these members of "the republic of silence and the night" face to face with the human condition in its starkest and most naked appearance. Obviously this republic featured human qualities which lay concealed and dormant in more normal conditions. Man is unmasked as irreducible freedom and transcendence.

The extreme situation of torture tests a man. But he always has the choice to talk or not, no matter how much the torturer might try and convince his victim that man is inhuman, that he must give in under pressure.[21] But even in the torture situation it is *possible* to demonstrate the freedom of man. The case of Henri Alleg exemplifies Sartre's viewpoint, for he showed that it was not necessary to take the torturer's view that man is constrained to give in and is not free in extreme situations. Alleg, tortured by paratroopers during the Algerian war, "naked, trembling with cold, tied to a plank still black and sticky from the vomit of earlier victims, reduced all

19. Sartre (1944), "Paris Alive: The Republic of Silence", *Atlantic Monthly*, CLXXIV, p. 39.
20. Ibid., p. 40.
21. Sartre (1958), "A Victory", Preface to Henri Alleg, *The Question*, p. 14.

these things to their pitiable true nature: they are comedies played by fools".[22] Alleg the victim "has conquered torture ... (T)he victim saves us in making us discover, as he has discovered himself, that we have the ability and the duty to undergo anything".[23] It only needs one man to save us from the fascination and vertigo we experience with the "whirlpool of inhumanity". For Sartre,

> When the victim wins, then it is goodbye to their absolute power, their lordship ... Because in the moment of victory one system of values is substituted for another; all it needs is that the torturers should become dizzy in their turn.[24]

According to Sartre, Alleg's difficult courage is as simple as it is exemplary, since he refused to enter into the games of his torturers. From the beginning Alleg *chose* to refuse all significance to torture.[25] He had made himself senseless to torture and showed that victory was possible in the most abject circumstances by turning the tables on the torturers by fighting them. Alleg's book on his experiences under torture affirms for Sartre that it is possible to win over tremendous forces by *scorning* them.[26] Sisyphean man, once again forced back on his resources may scorn the gods by revealing his freedom to himself and to those who would try and convince him that his freedom is a myth.[27] Sisyphus could not be more contemptuous.

A literature of extreme situations was created which depicted men living their condition to the limit and replaced a tradition of literature of average situations which had scarcely explored the human condition.[28] For those who lived the extremes however, humanity was to become

> a thin flame within them which they alone kept alive. It kept itself going in the silence which they opposed to their executioners. About them was nothing but the great polar night of the inhuman and of unknowingness, which they did not even *see*—which they guessed in the glacial cold which pierced them.[29]

22. Ibid., p. 16-17.
23. Ibid., p. 15.
24. Ibid., p. 27.
25. Sartre (1958), "La Réponse d'Henri Alleg", *Les Temps Modernes* 145, p. 1529.
26. Ibid., p. 1530.
27. Cf. Sartre (1946),"Materialism and Revolution" in *Literary and Philosophical Essays*, p. 221. Sartre (1947), *What is Literature*?, p. 138 for a contradictory view.
28. Sartre, *What is Literature*?, p. 163-64.
29. Ibid., p. 163.

This literature of extreme situations, far from making for hoplessness, revealed man's metaphysical freedom as much more than a thing, as radically divorced from the world of objects and as able to cope with any situation. The literature of extreme situations captured men at their starkest and yet most human level.

> Exile, captivity, above all death, which one easily shies from during happier times, were then our perpetual worry, and we were to learn that they were not avoidable accidents, not even constant or objective threats, but that we must discover in them our lot, our fate, the deepest source of our being.[30]

The extreme situations of man and the literature which so depicts him thus makes a metaphysician of him.

> For metaphysics is not a sterile discussion about abstract notions which have nothing to do with experience. It is a living effort to embrace from within the human condition in its totality.[31]

In this literature "it is always the whole man who is in question".[32] Thus the literature of extreme situations becomes a metaphysical literature about human freedom. The victim of the extreme situation can become a metaphysician, feeling his own freedom and repudiating outside determination: a man can never be entirely imprisoned. This is not to say that there are not many who would give in to their torturers in extreme situations. What Sartre is trying to show is that this is a *choice* whether the victim knows it or not. It is still possible to preserve a Sisyphean integrity in the worst situation, and further to become aware of insights of which we should not usually be aware.

Extreme situations do not occur only in war: madness is another way of experiencing man unmasked. In "The Room", Mme Darbédat remarks how illness sharpens the sensations.[33] M. Darbédat could see that Pierre the madman was analyzing himself too much, but did not know whether this was a cause or an effect of the sickness.[34] Sartre remarks in *Baudelaire* that "it must not be forgotten that as a result of their condition, Janet's patients frequently had metaphysical intuition where the normal person tries to hide from himself".[35] Baudelaire's *ennui* was itself a metaphysical

30. Sartre, "Paris Alive: The Republic of Silence", p. 39.
31. Sartre, *What is Literature?*, p. 164.
32. Ibid., p. 228.
33. Sartre (1938), "The Room" in *Intimacy*, p. 75.
34. *See* ibid., p. 84.
35. Sartre, *Baudelaire*, p. 31.

feeling which constituted his "interior landscape".[36] And of course, Hilbert in "Erostratus"—whose interior landscape is so schizophrenic—sees the world as an outsider, noting the absurdity of killing "all these people who are already dead".[37] *Nausea* explores the experiences of a similar man (the author!) who feels entirely cut off from the world of men and even of things. Sartre had always been fascinated with madness,[38] and if his works are not sufficient testimony to this, it can be noted that he himself went through periods of intense depression, even to the point of seeing lobsters following him.[39]

Sartre however, does not see madness as necessarily leading to an increased confrontation with *la condition humaine*. In *Altona*, Franz shuts himself up in a room and enacts a phantasy life worthy of the most paranoid schizophrenic precisely to *avoid* confronting reality. Indeed he chides Johanna for bringing the outside world into his room, his inner world: "My madness is falling in ruins. It was my refuge."[40] Madness can thus be a form of self-deception—for Franz, as for many of Laing's patients, it was a means of living in an otherwise unlivable world. When Franz finds the reality of a Germany that had lost the war and won the peace, and of the burgeoning prosperity of the family ship-building firm, he can no longer live. Yet at some level, Franz was aware of what he shut himself in from to hide from himself, for otherwise he would never have done so in the first place. His speeches to the court of crabs which he confesses are really men, are indeed very profound in their depiction of the state of man. Sartre's theory of the emotions understood madness as a magical defence against a threatening world,[41] and de Beauvoir recalls how Sartre refused to accept even physical illness[42] and one day decided that he was tired of being mad.[43]

But even where madness is used as a refuge in Sartre's work, it should not be forgotten that it reveals the human condition itself for Sartre. Franz has *seen* or *foreseen* the rise of Germany and cannot bear it, while many Germans live with it happily. In his room, the secrets of man "the flesh-eating beast" are disclosed— as indeed are those of the century itself. If we use madness as a refuge, it is only

36. Ibid., p. 28.
37. Sartre (1936), "Erostratus" in *Intimacy*, p. 126.
38. *See* S. de Beauvoir, *The Prime of Life*, p. 154.f
39. Ibid., p. 253.
40. Sartre (1969), *Altona*, p. 124.
41. Sartre (1939), *The Emotions: Outline of a Theory*.
42. de Beavoir,"Jean-Paul Sartre: Strictly Personal", *Harper's Bazaar*, and *The Prime of Life*, pp. 153-54.
43. Ibid., p. 265.

because we see too clearly. Thus the men who seek to escape "the human condition" through madness and those who seem to be plunged into madness are in an identical situation. Granted, they are "mad"—many among them would be the first to admit it. But their madness has placed them in an extraordinary situation which situates them outside the normal on the edge of the most comprehensive perceptions of the human condition. The madman is exiled, alone, without witnesses, recourse or reason. He is thus in a position to recognize what others take for granted or never think to challenge. He knows isolation in a godless world. His madness is a precondition for his metaphysics.

It is important to observe here that the boundaries of the disciplines of, say, psychology and philosophy simply do not exist for Sartre. Some psychologists might try and reduce or "explain" the ravings of a madman in terms of disturbed ego-functioning, and leave philosophical inquiry to be carried out by uncertifiable (or at any rate uncertified!) normal people. Sartre could simply answer that certain of the "ravings" were true, and madmen were in a privileged position to see, though they may not make use of this opportunity. Man even in madness is seen as freedom, as an irreducible and unexplainable nothingness. Similarly philosophy cannot be reduced to politics and history. "Existentialist" anguish as Sartre himself writes, can certainly be understood as "a historical and class phenomenon":

> Existentialism in its contemporary form appears with the decomposition of the bourgeoisie, and its origin is bourgeois. But that this decomposition can *disclose* certain aspects of the human condition and make possible certain metaphysical intuitions does not mean that these intuitions and this disclosure are illusions of the bourgeois consciousness or mythical representation of the situation.[44]

Even in his alleged conversion to Marxism, *Search for a Method* makes it abundantly clear that Marxism must incorporate existentialist perceptions without explaining them away.[45] But it is a sign of the age that these metaphysical intuitions of Sisyphean freedom are required to predominate. It is a condemnation of a system of life that forces man so far back in terms of his resources and power, that Sisyphean freedom becomes so relevant. For Sisyphus actually does live in a prison—the point is that he shows contempt for his gaolers who cannot possess his freedom under any circumstances. Madness

44. Sartre, *What is Literature*?, p. 230.
45. For example, Sartre, *Search for a Method*, p. 18.

too reveals the sickness of an age that makes such madness appropriate.

For Sartre, extreme situations are not qualitatively different from the normal ones—they reveal the inner nature of their normal situations by placing men into positions in which they can no longer hide the truth from themselves. They reveal the logic of everyday life which is normally truncated and mystified. For Sartre men feel they are nothing in everyday life and extreme situations provide them with the opportunity of finding out what they are in concrete tests.[46] Sartre's "average situations" are not ones in which people feel ontologically secure—they are situations in which they feel the very opposite: deep down there is a dread feeling of basic mistrust in themselves and their environment. Men are not sure of themselves, and Sartre's description of our being in terms of "the viscous"[47] involves a radical ontological insecurity for *everyone* "normal" or "mad". If we are characterized by such a radical ontological insecurity, extreme situations will show up what we "really are" as what we do in them assumes a fundamental importance. This can be taken as a sign of the times in which Sartre writes: men feel apathetic, cut adrift, insecure and afraid, and at the same time feel their lives to be determined by others and obscure social forces.[48]

Everything including man's freedom seems intangible in normal situations, but freedom can become real in extreme situations where action according to choice is necessary. Thus is unveiled man's fundamental quality of freedom which in an age of systematic intrusiveness into individual life becomes a proud last-ditch stand which is far more powerful than could hitherto have been imagined. We are radically divorced from the *être-en-soi*, (being-in-itself) and this is best seen when powerful forces seem to be trying to objectify man. Men can refuse to collude with those who believe the myth that men can be objectified—although they can (and often do) treat themselves as though they were objectifiable. For the early Sartre in particular, this is impossible, and belief in the status of man as an object is *mauvaise foi* (self-deception).[49]

Madness for Sartre is not seen as simple pathology, but is understood existentially in terms of relations between people; it is sometimes the only way out of living in an otherwise unlivable situation as in *Altona*—that is, madness is understood in terms of systems

46. For example, Sartre (1945), *Men Without Shadows*.
47. Sartre (1943), *Being and Nothingness*, Part Four, Ch. 1.
48. *See* ibid., Chs. 3,7.
49. Ibid., Part One, Ch. 2.

of social interaction. The person who goes mad in a sense chooses to do so for lack of possible alternatives as does Franz.[50] Thus there is an element of freedom, of choice. Although this freedom is a shrivelled one, it makes all the difference between man as subject who is involved in *praxis*, and man as object who undergoes a process. But a system in which such questions come to prominence is one in which the freedom to go mad is all that seems to be left: it indicates how far choice is restricted in the social systems.

So far I have argued that freedom for Sartre is of a Sisyphean kind in which all that seems available to men is an ultimate refusal of demands. Human reality is the basic datum for inquiry and this is equivalent to freedom for Sartre. This very emphasis on freedom indicates the problem of the *lack* of freedom in our age. We are conditioned by very powerful forces, but extreme situations can show us that we need not be entirely determined by them in any circumstance at all. We are stripped naked in these situations and certain metaphysical intuitions of our freedom can be thus disclosed. This freedom can be understood in broader systemic terms as a last-ditch stand against otherwise overwhelming forces—the torture victim may win over his torturers by dying without speaking; the madman uses his madness as a refuge in an otherwise unlivable situation. Freedom for Sartre is scarcely that of the Enlightenment—it represents freedom in chains, a statement that we are not *totally* imprisoned. The landscape of *Critique de la raison dialectique* personified in the world of Franz in *Altona* confirms this view.

Sartre contends that prison and play have been the favourite symbols of authors such as Pascal, Nietzsche and Kafka who have placed themselves outside the human condition so as to observe it.[51] This century has emphasized the prison to the virtual exclusion of authentic play which exists for its own sake. Kafka's seemingly endless rooms and corridors lead nowhere; Beckett's man is always waiting ... No one knows where his destiny will lead him. There is a radical divorce of intention and action and "loser wins" is the favourite game of Sartrean man. "Can we ever stop playing?" cries Hugo, distressed almost beyond words.[52] Man is doomed to never cease playing roles for he can never take on an authentic identity: he is condemned to be free. He can never achieve the solidity and massiveness of a rock without playing at doing so. Kean the actor, and

50. R.D. Laing (1960), *The Divided Self.*
51. Sartre, *Saint Genet*, p. 124.
52. Sartre (1948), *Crime Passionnel* (*Les Mains sales*) p. 75.

Kean the man mirror each other, and in the hall of mirrors which is man's existence, the actor and the man are indistinguishable.[53] (*Les Jeux sont faits—The Chips are Down*—is the title of one of Sartre's film scripts), but even in a wager with God, Sartrean man cheats—as Goetz did in *The Devil and the Good Lord*.[54]

Play, far from being the enjoyable and spontaneous expression of ourselves, is for Sartre an ontological necessity of the human reality of being-for-itself (*être-pour-soi*): it is our eternal absence from ourselves. That Sartre himself was confined in the prison of his grandfather's house until he was ten and never knew the company, much less enjoy the games of other children, is exceptional and could not be considered irrelevant, especially in the light of many other admissions in *Words*. In *The Age of Reason*, Mathieu is assailed by Marcelle for having acquired "the taste for self-analysis" in aiming to be "absolutely free". Mathieu explained to Marcelle as he did so often:

> "If I didn't try to get my life moving on my own account, I should think it just absurd to go on living ... It's not a vice. It's how I'm made."
> "Why aren't other people made like that if it isn't a vice?"
> "They are, only they don't know it."[55]

Sorbier in Sartre's play *Morts sans sépulture* (*Men Without Shadows*) remarks that everyone else does not know he is a coward.[56] The normal man in normal circumstances does not question his existence, he hides it from himself. He becomes caught up in games and lives his life in a world which is ineluctably a prison into which he is thrown and is of the Other's making; that is a situation into which he is plunged by the mere accident of being born at all, or at any rate born into a particular time and place. "Hell is other people", Garcin proclaimed in the closing lines of *Huis Clos (In Camera)*, and later Sartre explained that we, the living, live our lives in a "legitimate hell"[57] which is not of our choosing. Free in a world we do not choose—the world is a prison: once again freedom occurs in the context of imprisonment. Freedom is not the positive capacity to *be*; on the contrary it is the ability to refuse to be. Sartre's freedom is a negative one: it is not "freedom for" but "freedom from". This should be seen in the context of a situation of almost total domination.

53. *See* Sartre (1954), *Kean*.
54. Sartre (1951), *The Devil and the Good Lord*.
55. Sartre (1945), *The Age of Reason*, pp. 13-14.
56. Sartre, *Men Without Shadows*, p. 188.
57. Sartre, *Saint Genet*, p. 83.

Sartre's development constitutes a dialectic of freedom and determination. Certainly Orestes freely accepts and assumes the guilt of the Argyles and accursed, proudly exiles himself toward a new life. When Franz descends to the Other World, our world, and is encountered by his father, he gladly gives his guilt—and his life—to his father, and they finally suicide together as one. The Father's death would enshroud Franz's. The Father sees Franz as destined to impotence, crime and nothingness—he claims the guilt as his own, not Franz's. Yet the Father himself is slave to his own circumstances—in particular the Firm.[58]

From *Huis Clos* to *Altona*, the past gradually enters human reality, finally dominating it. "Childhood decides everything",[59] and the situation suppresses real choice.[60] There is no room for choice—and yet was there ever any in Sartre's work? Was it only an illusion? When Sartre writes of the "bitter-sweet madness" from which he has emerged,[61] it may partly be this illusion to which he is referring.

He had believed in the persuasive power of literature, its appeal to the freedom of its readers.[62] If the commitment of the writer was a weapon in the struggle against the forces of the night, it emerged as an illusion: literature is impotent. Whether it is the other who dominates one's world or scarcity, the real possibilities of authentic action seem remote. The freedom which takes us to the limits of the human condition seems a resigned one. If optimism, as Sartre says in one of his most "optimistic" works, is the belief that we do not suffer for nothing,[63] where are the real alternatives? If man is what he does rather than what he intends, where is freedom in a world in which our actions are doomed to backfire on us?

Our lives are dominated by macro-social forces, whether we know it or not. Before the war, Sartre was apolitical, yet one morning in 1939 all France recognized the political nature of things.[64] It was the war which brought Sartre into his view of commitment (*engagement*)—*Being and Nothingness*, published in 1943, reflects his life-long ontological preoccupations; *The Flies*, performed under the Occupation, admitted no freedom other than that of individual resistance—by Orestes leaving his kingdom! *Huis Clos*, while it purported to describe characters who were *dead*, in fact reflected the "living" categories of *Being and Nothingness*. As an individual, I de-

58. Sartre, *Altona*, pp. 159-63.
59. Sartre (1963), *Words*, p. 40.
60. Sartre (1960), "To Show, to Demonstrate", *Yale French Studies* 30, p. 41.
61. Sartre, *Words*, p. 157.
62. Sartre, *What is Literature*?, p. 36.
63. Sartre, *Saint Genet*, p. 557.
64. Sartre (1955), "... Said Jean-Paul Sartre", *Yale French Studies* 16, p. 4.

pend on the Other's recognition; and yet I cannot control him without his collusion—and this can only involve a pseudo-recognition. Inwardly I am, to use Laing's phrase, "ontologically in-secure" since there is no foundation to my existence. This lack of foundation constitutes my distinction from the world of objects.

The terms that denote our existence—"condemned to be free", "abandoned", "without excuse", "without appeal", "lack", "nothingness", "viscous", "oozing", "jelly-like", "nauseous", and more lately "violence", "terror", "scarcity"—are all negative.[65] When Sartre writes of religion as his "missed vocation",[66] he neglects to explicitly point out that its substitute was literature. For Sartre, man was condemned to miss the plenitude of being: by the desire to be God, and in his hunger for the absolute, man was doomed to deprivation.[67] An anecdote has been told that in a discussion between Sartre and Marcel, Marcel had said that he *believed* in God's existence. Sartre retaliated that not only did he *believe*, but that he *knew* that God did not exist. Humorists wondered whether God himself had revealed his non-existence to Sartre.[68] This dialogue with the silent partner who does not exist constitutes Sartre's universe. Of course Sartre protests that God's non-existence leaves men to create and adhere to their own values. "Existentialism is nothing else but an attempt to draw the full conclusions from a consistently atheistic position."[69]

But this absolute denial of the absolute is a sign of the need for it. Why? Perhaps because otherwise there is no possibility of salvation at all. We are all prisoners condemned to a life sentence in Hell. Manichaeism supposed the co-presence of the Devil and of the Good Lord. Sartre is a Manichaeist without God: evil is irreducible and good does not exist. Goetz' resignation to an earthly salvation is scarcely a happy one:

> Never fear, I shall not flinch. I shall make them hate me, because I know no other way of loving them. I shall give them orders; since I have no other way of obeying. I shall remain alone with an empty sky over my head, since I have no other way of being among men. There is this war to fight, and I will fight it.[70]

The empty sky signifies God's absence, the rest seems to signify a

65. *See* M. Cranston, "Sartre and Violence", *Encounter*, July 1967.
66. Sartre, *Words*, p. 65.
67. Sartre, *Being and Nothingness*, p. 784.
68. R. Jolivet, *Sartre ou la théologie de l'absurde*, p. 9.
69. Sartre (1946), *Existentialism and Humanism*, p. 58.
70. Sartre, *The Devil and the Good Lord*, p. 149.

Sisyphean type defiance of the Devil, of the Hell that is our situation. Goetz is not Sartre himself, but who Sartre would like to be![71] Sartrean man is the willing slave of neither the Devil nor the Good Lord. But he is an unwilling slave to his condition which is defined in terms of evil and damnation. He is Camus' Sisyphus who scorns the gods who have punished him by eternally involving him in the most useless and arduous tasks in a most useless eternal life. Yet the gods could not take scorn and even joy from Sisyphus.[72] The rock is pushed up only to roll down: most of Sartre's situations are set up only to find later how useless they were in the first place. The optimism of a Sisyphus can only lie in the notice the gods take of his supreme contempt for them. His suffering is not in vain if the gods are cowed by his inner refusal to accept the condition in which they have placed him.

Sartrean freedom can then be seen not only in the context of the world as a prison without bars, but also as a prison without rations. Man is inherently deprived of the allness a God might confer on him by man's inner constitution as a nothingness—it is a privation. Further, this prison is an earthly hell without the possibility of heaven or even purgatory, since God is dead. We are damned and condemned to a frustrating freedom in a world in which evil prevails. Perhaps Sartre is echoing the classical view of the relation of evil and privation. In any case man seems doomed to continue in a Sisyphean form what the evil gods have ordained, and at the same time have the consciousness that Sisyphus has of the absurdity of his endeavours. However, while a person might outwardly comply with the hellish demands made on him by his social systems, he retains an inner core which can still say "No".

Freedom is not only a refusal in a prison situation, but also can be seen as using outward conformity through role-playing to satisfy the outer demands, yet keeping the inner self distant and distinct from the roles it plays in the world to which man is condemned. The body and the world act to imprison the "soul", but the soul also keeps its own identity by not being the body or the world, while it keeps in negative relation with them. Through role-playing, a person can keep the world away, just as Sisyphus performed the tasks required of him without submitting inwardly to the gods. Sisyphean man has the notice of the evil "gods". Sartre's godless universe is evil,

71. "He was the perfect embodiment of the man of action as Sartre conceived him. 'I made Goetz do what I was unable to do'." de Beauvoir, *Force of Circumstance*, p. 254.
72. Camus, *The Myth of Sisyphus*.

perhaps because it is lacking in the allness that would bring good, in the fullness of being itself. But without God, being becomes repulsive.[73] A Manichaeism without God rules Sartrean man who is in constant dialogue with the silent partner—the non-existent God. Sartrean man has certainly missed out on ontological security! He seems radically divorced from a place in the world around him and seems to be able to exercise little or no control over it. His freedom is the freedom to refuse to be controlled explicitly, yet he must act in a world in which his choices seem conditioned for him, and in which he seems in fact to be controlled by obscure forces of which he is unaware that affect his existence.[74]

The resignation of Sisyphean man to earthly damnation stands in contrast to the optimism of a Prometheus who brought to man the fire Zeus had hidden and is known as the creator of man. According to Marx, the profession of philosophy is that of Prometheus: "In simple words, I hate the pack of gods." It is philosophy's

> own aphorism against all divine and earthly gods who do not acknowledge human self-consciousness as the highest divinity. It allows no rivals ... Prometheus is the most eminent saint and martyr in the philosophic calendar.[75]

There are of course important similarities between Prometheus and Sisyphus; both are tricksters, both have been enchained and both hate the gods. So far Sartre would agree that this is the lot of man. But where Sisyphus acknowledges the gods as the highest divinity against whom he is contemptuous, Prometheus makes humanity itself the highest divinity, hating all who would mystify the situation. While Sisyphus will never be ruled by the gods altogether, Prometheus defiantly asserts himself.

The difference between Sartre's Sisyphean framework and that of a Prometheus can be described shortly in the cry of Epicurus: "The blasphemous is not he who scorns the gods or the masses, but those who adhere to the idea that the masses create the gods".[76] Sartre's austere stoicism and stern optimism[77] are of the former kind and not of the latter, for Sartre accepts God's non-existence as an absence, a deprivation, and man's actions are doomed to be gestures: existence

73. Sartre (1938), *Nausea*.
74. Sartre, *What is Literature*?, p. 157. G. Bateson, *Steps to an Ecology of Mind*, p. 410.
75. K. Marx, *The Difference Between the Democratean and Epicurean Philosophy of Nature* in N.D. Livergood; *Activity in Marx's Philosophy*, p. 62.f
76. Cited in idem.
77. Sartre, *Existentialism and Humanism*, p. 42.

is described in negative terms, and our freedom is what we can do in very limited conditions—man can always say "No". This constitutes his irreducibility to the natural order, and he can be proud of the resistance he puts up against the powers that be.[78]

Promethean man, however, hates the pack of gods, not because they deprive him, but because he does not want them to exist at all. Sisyphean man is condemned; Promethean man creates and overcomes the pre-existing situation.

Our epoch has been one in which our terrible freedom has been exposed to us: it is a burden we do not want to bear. It is interesting that the primary category of freedom in Sartre is one which is seen so willingly to deny its own existence through deceiving itself. Sartre's concern with self-deception is important only in an era where self-deception and the wish to deceive oneself is the rule. Stripped of our deceptions, our inner core of freedom is revealed. This disaster is transformed into a triumph. In spite of all we can be aware of ourselves as not entirely determined—there is a precious something (nothingness!) that no one can take away from us. We shall not submit, nor shall we enter with our souls the games the human condition imposes. We may seem to be playing along in roles, but we are not really. Sartre had discovered something new in *la réalité humaine*. Sisyphus is not beaten after all; he has a distinct identity. "When people speak to me about freedom," Sartre used to say, "it is as if they were speaking about myself."[79] According to Merleau-Ponty, Sartre

> identifies himself with that transparency and that agility which is not of the world and which as he has written, makes men "mortal". That is an intuition from which one may go forward but cannot turn back—and which those who wish to remain asleep will always find disagreeable.[80]

This intuition of freedom is in the Cartesian tradition with which

78. Another Greek myth is relevant to this myth of Sisyphus. Daedalus fashioned two pairs of wings for himself and Icarus and the larger pair was threaded together while the smaller pair was held together by wax. "My son be warned," Daedalus told Icarus. "Neither soar too high lest the sun melt the wax; nor swoop too low, lest the feathers be wetted by the sea ... Follow me closely." Yet when Icarus had disobeyed his father's instructions and had flown towards the sun, the wax of his wings had melted and he fell into the sea and was drowned in it. But for Sartre God the Father is absent, and Icarus abandoned can follow what path he will, but the result is the same—disaster. *See* R. Graves, *The Greek Myths*, *Vol.* I, pp. 312-13.
79. Cited by M. Merleau-Ponty, *Sense and Non-sense*, p. 47.
80. Ibid., p. 47.

Sartre aligns himself,[81] but is not a purely intellectual intuition. It is the radical *experience* of not being thing-like. Pablo in "The Wall" does not care a rap for Spain when confronted with the imminence of the wall of death. Lucie, in *Morts sans sépulture*, refuses to talk under torture not out of her love for Jean, but so as to win over the torturers. As with the Alleg case discussed above, the torturers would have us believe that any man will talk after more or less torture, but the horror of the torture chamber is the spark which will not be put out. Even the torturers cannot eliminate the *pour-soi*. This is the situation in which Sartre finds himself to be "optimistic". According to Sartre, it is not so much the pessimism of existentialism, but the sternness of its optimism that irks people.[82] If man is by nature evil, then that cannot be helped. If we are entirely doomed, then we might as well give in. Sartre's "optimism" amounts to the view that if it is really *possible* for any man to die under torture and say nothing, that a man does not have to give in, that we are, after all, still free in prison!

So far then, Sartre's Sisyphean resigned acceptance of damnation can be seen—and this stands in stark contrast to the Promethean vision of the positive view of an open future. The question is then why this Sisyphean freedom is the one that Sartre sees as the only real one now—for Sartre certainly does not have a Promethean approach. It would seem that this is because the Sisyphean one is the only real possibility this century since we are irrevocably trapped in our earthly hell which is so overwhelming that no authentic move towards a good society seems really possible. This is a sad comment on the state of the world, and a Sisyphean freedom is better than none at all. That is, it maintains the last vestiges of ourselves as having any identity of our own at all.

But for Sartre most of our choices are determined whether we know it or not. Even Sisyphean freedom seems to be at stake where we are not even aware of the range of choices, where the choices are very complex, or where we are completely mystified about our condition.

The prison gates do not open with the *Critique de la raison dialectique*: we all live under the terror of the group under the reign of scarcity.[83] Nothing could be more terrible for man according to Sartre than

81. *See* Sartre's statement cited in M. Contat and M. Rybalka, *Les Ecrits de Sartre*, p. 108.
82. Sartre, *Existentialism and Humanism*, p. 42.
83. Sartre (1960), *Critique de la raison dialectique*.

> an intelligent flesh-eating species, capable of understanding and outwitting human intelligence, and whose prime aim lies in the destruction of man. This species is obviously our own, comprehending itself in each individual through the intermediary of others in an environment dominated by scarcity.[84]

Our external and internal landscapes are remarkably similar. The individual who formerly could preserve some integrity against the Other finds himself enmeshed in a web of mediations he cannot possibly control or understand. If satisfactory relations between two people who are not situated historically are impossible, how possible are authentic relations among people in groups who are mediated historically? The individual is virtually impotent in the face of all others who exist now and who have conditioned his own past. What we are depends on our childhood, "completely deprived or completely endowed, we are lost".[85]

Our childhood may leave us some choice. Genet, for example, was not only the child brought up by peasants, but had an identity somewhere in the city in a foundling registry. What was a narrow area of choice in the early Sartre is narrowed very much further as the power of the past and of the macro-social context widens. Sartre was aware of this even in 1947 when he wrote that from 1930 on, "obscure and collective forces" had in fact governed peoples' minutest gestures, "the most private circumstances seemed to reflect the state of the whole world". And the secret of these gestures "lay ahead of us in a catastrophe to which our names would be attached".[86] In 1960, he writes:

> The social field is full of acts with no author, of constructions without constructor. If we rediscover in man his veritable humanity—that is, his power to make History by pursuing his own ends—*then* in a period of alienation, we shall see that the non-human is presented with all the appearances of the human and that the "collectives", perspectives of flight across men, retain in themselves the finality which characterizes human relations ... The indissoluble unity of these "apparatus", these monstrous constructions with no author in which man loses himself and which forever escape him, with their rigorous functioning, their reversed finality (which should be called, I think, a *counter-finality*), with their pure or "natural" necessities and the furious struggle of alienated men—this indissoluble unity must appear to every inquirer who wants to comprehend the social world.[87]

84. Sartre, *Critique de la raison dialectique*, p. 208, translated and cited in P. Thody, *Sartre: A Biographical Introduction*, p. 123.
85. Sartre (1961), "Merleau-Ponty" in *Situations*, p. 228.
86. Sartre, *What is Literature?*, p. 157.
87. Sartre, *Search for a Method*, pp. 163-64.

The vagabonds without authors are so far out of control that they militate against the very ends towards which they were intended. They are irreducible and enhance our alienation still further. The flesh-eating species has produced a machine it can no longer control, and which assumes greater and greater power over our lives. The theme is familiar. Earlier in the century, Kafka had written of the rising technical-bureaucracy which Weber described as an "iron cage". More recently, Marcuse has described a "one-dimensional" society which has become self-regulating and in which opposition is assimilated as testifying to the justice of that society.

Formal rationality is appropriate to a society in which subject and object have achieved a unity which aims toward the perpetuation of a life which is best defined in calculable terms. The agents of oppression seem to be liberating us from their power. The communications media level importance and triviality in an entertaining whole.

Sartre's monstrous constructions rule the world in their counter-finality. Especially in an age where the family is breaking down and people are far more other-directed and manipulable than previously, the child experiences far more than just his family. "He lives also—in part through the family—the collective landscape which surrounds him. It is again the generality of his class which is revealed to him in this individual experience."[88] The world Sartre describes is one of myriads of intertwining systems of socialization which leave the individual virtually no room for choice at all. And where there seems to be a choice, there is no guarantee of the end being achieved. As the Father says in *Altona*, trying to win is "the surest way of losing".[89] *Huis Clos* was about dead characters who were forever what they were at their death; *Altona* is about people who are forever what they are at their birth. The earth is now hell and the devil is mankind; there is no exit.

This reinforces the earlier theme about freedom being the ability to inwardly refuse; our world is such that this type of freedom—what in former times would have been considered a caricature of freedom—is highlighted because that is all that we can be sure of. But even here, freedom somehow evaporates, absorbed into social matrices beyond comprehension. Man is always involved in praxis, but it is so alienated that he does not understand what he is doing, nor even often enough that he is doing it at all.[90] We may not be aware of our freedom since the complexity of group mystification is

88. Sartre, *Search for a Method*, p. 79.
89. Sartre, *Altona*, p. 150.
90. R.D. Laing and D.G. Cooper (1964), *Reason and Violence: A Decade in Sartre's Philosophy 1950-1960*, p. 112ff, 172ff.

so great. Formerly the choices seemed reasonably simple and man could assert his Sisyphean freedom against the forces which, while they were overwhelming, were nonetheless visible. When the past and group mystifications enter Sartre's field and action is so alienated as to have a reversed finality about it, individual freedom comes to be seen as alien, yet collective freedom is still further impossible. Man has become lost in the now autonomous systems he has created through his collective practice, consciously and unconsciously. The systemic consequences of a collection of individual or organizational actions were not considered and the consequences of our actions have gone right out of our control and exert control over us—the worst forms being where we are controlled yet do not realize it. This is the situation in which individual "freedom" can only be understood in terms of the social totality in which the individual lives. Indeed, the individual does not exist; he is so dominated by micro- and macro-social systems of the past and the present. Individual freedom is thus seen as impossible.

We must look to the *epoch* as the primary totality, such is the immensity and intensity of the individual's systemic existence. He can only be understood as almost totally conditioned by the results of the intermeshing of the systems he lives whether or not he is aware of them. If the individual has disappeared into the conditioning systems of his epoch, those systems will also be evident in individual biography. They will incarnate themselves in the individual as the individual will incarnate his epoch. Of course these internalizations, the externalizations of these and their reinternalizations are no simple matter, and each individual lives the same or different sets of systems in a different way. Yet the general systemic *framework* in which we live them is the same, for our problematic is the whole which pervades all of its parts. Sartre writes:

> If the truth is one, we must as Gide said of God, seek it not elsewhere but everywhere. Each social product and each attitude—from the most private to the most public—are its allusive incarnations. An anecdote reflects an entire era as much as the substance of a political constitution.[91]

We are so alienated that not only can I not say "I am I", but the freest people can say only "I exist". But this is already too much. "For the others I suggest that they use formulae such as 'I am Himself' or 'I am so-and-so in *person*'." Sartre keeps away from such impersonations of people as he does not like "inhabited souls". He maintains, however, that

91. Sartre, "Merleau-Ponty", p. 241.

> if you suffer a perpetual absence at your very core, then you can live this absence as that of any other. That other will never be more absent than you are, for the way in which he is not himself, ... the way in which you are not you, and the way in which you are not he do not differ appreciably.[92]

Thus we are alienated whether inhabited or not—for the "me" is as other as the "you" or the "himself" is. Again we have an absence at the core which might be considered "freedom", but is in fact quite strictly nothing at all, an absence. In a way we might consider that we are living in "extreme situations" all the time since there is nothing which is ours, and we are always under threat of engulfment. We are not our bodies, actions, expectations—these belong to the systems we live. We are cut off from them, and all that is left as ours is an absence. This is the position the schizoid occupies in Laing's *The Divided Self*.[93] It is a situation of total alienation. Being absent at our core, we are the same as anybody else is. For the rest, it is now the social whole that determines our existence. Writing of his relationship with Merleau-Ponty, Sartre concludes:

> Each of you may blame who you will. In any case, we weren't really guilty, so little in fact, that sometimes all I can see in our adventure was its necessity. That is the way men live in our time. That is the way they love. Badly.[94]

According to Sartre, there are today only two modes of speaking of oneself: "the third person singular or the first person plural. We must first know how to say 'we' in order to say 'I' ".[95] We are each a "unique anybody",[96] and Sartre himself writes to express the period through himself since he is like everyone else. In writing *Words*, he was not only concerned with the meaning of his life, but wanted to "recall the rather curious history of a generation".[97]

For Sartre, Kierkegaard had discovered that the universal enters the singular in history to the extent that the singular instantiates the universal.[98] In his recent study of Flaubert, Sartre writes that since a man is never an individual, it would be better to call him a "universal singular" who is totalized, and thus universalized by his epoch. He also retotalizes it in his reproducing it as a singular. He is universal by the singular universality of human history and singular

92. Sartre, *Saint Genet*, pp. 83-84.
93. *See* Ch. 5.
94. Sartre, "Merleau-Ponty", p. 326.
95. Sartre (1958), "Of Rats and Men" in *Situations*, p. 370.
96. Ibid., p. 368.
97. Sartre, Interview with Oliver Todd.
98. Sartre (1964), "L'Universel singulier" in *Kierkegaard vivant*.

by the universalizing singularity of his projects.[99]

Each of us is a man of his time—"a man is his whole period as a wave is the whole sea".[100] Sartre the writer writes what he feels and is not enslaved by political considerations. He constantly points out that he is a writer and not a politician,[101] and further that it is the duty of the writer "to show, to demonstrate, to unveil hoaxes, to dissolve myths and fetishes with a small bath of critical acid".[102] Sartre aims himself at reaching the "profundity of the lived",[103] and at describing "lived experience",[104] his own as well as that of others. The writers Sartre is interested in bear such remarkable similarities to himself however for this to be coincidental.[105] Through self-analysis carried out often enough through others, Sartre touches the mood of our time, and recreates it for us—or rather we, in reading him, recreate it for ourselves. As he says "reading involves rewriting"[106] and this is certainly true of Sartre's readings! But it does not make it the less "accurate" since in reflecting himself, he is reflecting his time and ours.

As each of us incarnates all of mankind, or at least our contemporary culture, the enemy becomes our twin brother—"our image in the mirror. These evil men are as necessary to good men as whores are to decent men", Sartre writes graphically.[107] And if every man is all of man, the black sheep Genet "must be only a pebble or must be me".[108] There is little doubt in Sartre's mind that Genet is not a pebble, and so finally we must look into the mirror that Genet holds up to us and see ourselves as guilty.[109] For Sartre, even the iron curtain is only a mirror—each half of the world reflects the other half. "He who condemns today must know that our situation tomorrow will force him to do worse than what he is condemning", Sartre wrote in his *Reply to Albert Camus*.[110] Perhaps we may find some freedom

99. Sartre (1971), *L'Idiot de la famille*, Preface.
100. Sartre, "To Show, To Demonstrate", p. 43.
101. *See* for example, Sartre: "... Said Jean-Paul Sartre", p. 5, *Playboy* interview with Sartre, p. 166.
102. Sartre, "To Show, To Demonstrate", p. 42.
103. Sartre, *Search for a Method*, p. 145.
104. "The conception of 'lived experience' marks my change since *L'Etre et le néant*", Sartre ( 1969), "Itinerary of a Thought", *New Left Review 58*, p. 50.
105. F. Jeanson, *Sartre par lui-même*, pp. 74-75. P. Thody, *Sartre: a Biographical Introduction*, pp. 19-20. T. Molnar, *Sartre: Ideologue of Our Time*, p. 13. M. Cranston, *Sartre*, Ch. 9.
106. Sartre, "To Show, To Demonstrate", p. 43.
107. Sartre, *Saint Genet*, p. 30.
108. Ibid., p. 587.
109. Ibid., p. 599.
110. Sartre (1952), "Reply to Albert Camus" in *Situations*, p. 86.

through demystifying ourselves and our epoch and realize that *we* do evil and it is *we* who blame scapegoats for this. Our existence can be seen as a vast system of mirrors, reflecting and refracting each other so far that we see and put in others what we do not like in ourselves, and these others often play the roles into which they are thrust. Both us and them are lost[111] and freedom is a myth if we have no real idea of our own identity. Perhaps we should try to regain a sense of who we are by the study of the systems each of us lives.

A method for studying the situation today is that of studying biography heuristically.[112] In the notion of biography which is the point of insertion of man in his culture[113] Sartre employs a psychoanalytic method in looking at childhood,[114] but at no stage is involved in reductionism. The dialectic

> follows the reverse procedure. It surpasses by conserving, but the terms of the surpassed contradiction cannot account for either the transcending itself or the subsequent synthesis; on the contrary, it is the synthesis which clarifies them and which enables us to understand them ... It is the work or the act of the individual which reveals to us the secret of his conditioning.[115]

We are in constant process of surpassing the given,[116] and it is important for us in understanding or comprehending a person to see him as signifying, as reaching towards the future.[117]

What has always interested Sartre is not so much human nature as the human condition we live.[118] Thus what interests Sartre in Genet is not so much the conditioning processes he underwent, as his overcoming of them. The interesting question for Sartre is not why people under certain bad conditions become criminals, madmen, workers and so on, but why some do *not*. Genet is a perfect case. Instead of adopting the role he was flung into—through his conditions—he transcended his condition by the writing of *Our Lady of the Flowers*. Such a transformation is understandable, according to Sartre, ultimately only in terms of freedom, although Marxist and psychoanalytic theories may aid in reconstructing the life.[119]

111. *See* R.D. Laing (1967), "Us and Them" in *The Politics of Experience and the Bird of Paradise*.
112. Sartre, *Search for a Method*, p. 135.
113. Ibid., p. 62.
114. Ibid., p. 60.
115. Ibid., pp. 151-52.
116. Ibid., p. 100.
117. Ibid., pp. 152-53.
118. Sartre, *Existentialism and Humanism*, pp. 45-46.
119. Sartre, *Saint Genet*, p. 449.

Bettleheim observes that psychoanalytic studies of the personalities of great men such as Leonardo, Beethoven, Goethe and Swift, have typically focussed on pathology. "But the real enigma is not the psychopathology, but the creative contributions." Freud, for example, "sheds no light on the problem of why Leonardo became a great inventor and artist when the same experiences might have led to empty scribbling or purposeless gadgeteering in others". Such biographies "present us with fascinating sidelights on the lives of their heroes, but fail to make at all plainer why their work, that is their positive contribution to mankind, took place". The biographies show us that "psychoanalysis is the best method for uncovering and understanding the hidden man, but by no means an especially good method for understanding man in his entirety".[120]

Psychoanalysis can thus illuminate the conditions in which a life is undertaken as can a sociological investigation. But finally, at least in some cases, freedom may manifest itself. It is precisely in the most horrific circumstances that Henri Alleg succeeded in shouting out to his torturers, "You can come back with your magneto, I await you: I am not afraid of you".[121] In his *Temps Modernes* editorial, Sartre writes that Alleg's book is the first "optimistic" book on the Algerian War.[122]

Similarly, ridiculed by his fellow-prisoners, Genet writes *Our Lady* in a cell. Sartre writes in *Saint Genet* that Genet's story is one of liberation. Indeed his ten years of writing are the equivalent of a "psychoanalytic cure".[123] It should be obvious by now that Sartre sees Genet's condition as our own.

> Today God is dead, even in the heart of the believer, and art becomes an anthropodicy ... There is an ethic of Beauty: it requires of us a kind of demiurgic stoicism; optimism without hope, acceptance of Evil as a condition of total unity, affirmation of human creative reality over and above its failures in a universe that crushes it; assumption by freedom of suffering, faults and death; we must will being as though we had made it.[124]

Optimism then becomes "the affirmation not that man is or can be happy, but simply that he does not suffer for nothing ... We find here again the game loser wins".[125]

120. B. Bettleheim, *The Informed Heart*, p. 34.
121. Sartre, "La Réponse d'Henri Alleg", p. 1529. (My translation)
122. Ibid., p. 1530.
123. Sartre, *Saint Genet*, p. 544.
124. Ibid., p. 497.
125. Ibid., p. 557.

The well-known statement of Orestes that "life begins on the other side of despair" is given more meaning in an article Sartre wrote in 1944:

> True optimism begins with despair, the optimism of a man who expects nothing, who knows that he has no rights and that nothing is due to him, who rejoices in relying on himself alone and working for the good of all.[126]

Yet the other side of this "optimism" about man's ultimate freedom, is dramatically characterized by Mathieu:

> There had been, and forever would be, that cold glare upon those stones under the black sky; the absolute, forever: the absolute without cause or sense or purpose, without past or future, save a gratuitous, fortuitous splendid permanence. "I am free", he said suddenly and his joy shrivelled into horror.[127]

For Mathieu, "nothing can ever grasp or absorb me. Outside the world, outside the past, outside myself; freedom is exile, and I am condemned to be free".[128]

In our age, according to Sartre, where "all is violence"[129] and where the "universe remains dark, we are animals struck by catastrophe".[130] Sartre claims that his "optimism" is on the side of those who think that the world *could* be better, where socio-economic ills are alleviated.[131] But the metaphysical ills remain, and Sartre's development consists partly at least in his abandoning the hope of formulating a morality.[132] Sartre admits that he has changed, but "as everyone changes, within a permanence".[133]

Even here, however, it is difficult to account for or grasp the freedom Sartre attributes to our inner core. No methodology seems adequate. Sartre often goes back to the "original choice" of the person to become a writer—this occurs round the age of seven or eight.

But this itself seems a little arbitrary. In *Les Mains sales*, Hugo returns after spending years in gaol wondering why he killed Hoederer. All he knows is that he fired the shots. In an attempt to understand, Olga asks him to begin his story at the beginning. Hugo

126. Sartre in *Action*, 1944. Translated and cited in M.-A. Burnier, *Choice of Action*, p. 25.
127. Sartre (1945), *The Reprieve*, p. 299.
128. Ibid., p. 308.
129. Sartre (1947), "The Responsibility of the Writer", in *Reflections on Our Age*, p. 82.
130. Sartre (1964), "A Long Bitter-Sweet Madness", *Encounter XXII*, p. 61.
131. Ibid., p. 62.
132. Idem.
133. Ibid., p. 63.

replies:

> The beginning? You know it as well as I do. Anyway, was there ever a beginning? You can begin the story in forty-three when Louis sent for me. Or you can begin it the year before when I joined the Party, or before that when I was born.[134]

The beginning and the end seem frighteningly outside our control, and any methodology will be relative. We can only look backward to find some of the factors leading us to making our choices: and even this is seen through the prisms of our present projects and visions. We do not know very often whether our choices are "free" or not. Indeed Sartre wonders whether he himself became a writer simply "in the sole and mad hope of pleasing my grandfather".[135] His own autobiography cannot be taken at face-value. Is he describing what actually happened in his childhood or how he sees his childhood today looking backwards towards it, and if the latter, has he moulded his themes to suit his later existential psychoanalytic viewpoint? The description may well be an interpretation.[136] Of course, not only is our view of the past governed to quite an extent by our own socialization, but in terms of what we now want from it for the future. Sartre is no impartial, dead, objective ideal observer, for no one can be. In his preface to Jeanson's book on the moral problem in Sartre, Sartre compliments Jeanson for not treating the work of a living author as if he were dead and was finished forever.[137] But the possibilities for interpretation of a dead author's writings are as wide as the interpretations of the period itself and of the interpreter himself.

Sartre will always go down fighting, but the problematic or permanence within which his work structures itself remains basic. Certainly there is a dynamic, and it is in this that the subject lives. But the basic structures of the given overwhelming reality ultimately triumph and inhabit the individual. In a sense it is not very valuable to search for freedom in biography, yet it is important to realize that all is praxis however alienated it may be. It is another question entirely as to whether an unalienated praxis might overcome the condition in which praxis is seen as process. From what has been said so far, this possibility in fact does not exist for Sartre. In other words, our actions are irreducible to those of machines, but we are so dis-

134. Sartre, *Crime Passionnel*, p. 17.
135. Sartre, *Words*, p. 103.
136. J.P. Fell, "Sartre's *Words': an Existential Self-Analysis", Psychoanalytic Review* 55, p. 430.
137. Sartre (1947), Lettre-Préface to F. Jeanson; *Le Problème moral et la pensée de Sartre*.

tant from ourselves and our conditions—which are themselves so enveloping and dominating—that we see our practice as not our own. Even if we were to see it as our own, we could not predict the consequences. Simple categories of freedom, optimism, salvation and so on, cannot be instantiated in the modern world. All we can do is to try and see what is happening in our names before our eyes and wrest something of ourselves from domination in our distancing ourselves from it. If we cannot recognize freedom in our actions since they seem to have no authors in a logic of their own, we may try at least to define the character of our time through the biography of an individual. Under the massive weight of a truly alienated praxis, freedom and individuality seem irretrievably lost. The man disappears into the vastness of his time.

Perhaps the bastard alone can hold on in some measure—this may be Sartre's "optimism". Goetz says—"We *are* nothing and *have* nothing. Every infant born in wedlock can inherit the earth without paying."[138] Yet God the Father is now dead, and man today is abandoned, thrown, condemned, without excuse and without appeal. This is so, even if many do not know it. The bastard is in a privileged position since he sees the world from outside and owes nothing to it. He is free for nothing, perhaps because he does not feel there is anything which can be his. He lives in an extreme situation and is lucid because he can see what is going on without being involved—and cannot hide it from himself as the rest of men can. As Jeanson says, lucidity is the property of the consciousness which discovers its detachment; it is that of the Actor.

Sartre is the ideal bastard because his bastardy is not "the result of accident resulting from badly supervised coitus, nor is it subject to legal review or remedy". He was totally accepted, so totally legitimate that he knew no sense of property at all.'[139] There was no sense of being a person who owned anything—Sartre was never accepted as a person, but as a model boy. It was the model boy who was legitimate. The facade, not the real young Sartre was accepted by his family. He did not belong in his family or to the world—only his roles did. The young Sartre was abandoned as a person who had to fend for himself like the young Genet. Like Genet, who was never given anything without some sort of obligation, Sartre tried to make up for his having been given everything. He had no sense of personal autonomy or acceptance; thus favours done him involved reciprocal obligations and guilt, because he felt he was given things he did not

138. Sartre, *The Devil and the Good Lord*, p. 33.
139. Jeanson, "Hell and Bastardy", *Yale French Studies* 30, pp. 6-7.

deserve. The young Sartre felt he had to be the person others wanted him to be, to live up to their expectations. Thus he removed himself further from them because it was not the real Sartre who was being accepted, but the false impostor. This could only increase his alienation and feeling of not belonging, since he felt the real Sartre was being rejected and abandoned. The vision of a world in which man can "inherit the earth without paying" can only occur where man is legitimate—as he was during the time of Goetz, centuries ago.

But now bastardy seems man's fundamental condition. We live in a fatherless society, in which mother has not been able to give us a sense of autonomy, and in which we seem to have no fundamental right to a self-justifying and rich life we can call our own. We are articulate, we can see our position, but are powerless to do anything about it. Our hunger for the absolute will never be satisfied we know now with certainty. We are alone now and if "every epoch discovers an aspect of the condition of humanity",[140] this age exhibits the most what man has made of himself in its most lucid and horrific form. If an epoch, like a man, is a future in the Sartrean scheme of things,[141] it is one we shall never grasp as both the present and the future are out of our control. We shall never feel that the world we live in is *ours*, belongs to us, since it is so alienated. We are doomed to a reversed finality in our actions—whether individual or collective—so far have things gotten out of hand.

For Sartre, the only freedom that seems possible is of the Sisyphean type of inward refusal since we live condemned to a life sentence in the earthly prison without bars which is our hell. It is a sign of our age that this type of freedom seems the only possible one. Extreme situations can show men their freedom, since in ordinary circumstances they do not challenge their conceptions, yet they do not feel ontologically secure either. In Sisyphean freedom, we can see and confront our condition and turn our disaster into triumph: we can refuse *total* determination. But gradually for Sartre, both the past and the group entered the scene so far as to dominate it. We are determined, whether we know it or not, by the mystified systems we live. Certainly we are engaged in praxis, but it is so mystified and alienated that we cannot recognize ourselves in it. We act in ignorance and the results of our actions come back on us in the unintended consequences of a reversed finality. We are free, but we do not know when or in what circumstances we are. Freedom becomes a lie because man is lost in the now autonomous systems of monstrous constructions he has created. The individual disappears into his time

140. Sartre (1945), "The Case for Responsible Literature", *Partisan Review XII*, p. 308.
141. Ibid., p. 307.

as a universal singular and a demystification of individual biography may reveal the secrets of the individual and his time as the systems he lives. Biography presupposes a degree of freedom and cannot be reduced to psychoanalytical or sociological categories. Ultimately, it can be explained in terms of freedom in the case of people who are conditioned *not* fulfilling the roles into which they are thrust—people such as Genet who transformed himself through freely writing. The task of the writer is to unveil and demystify reality; to show ourselves to ourselves so that we might be able to act more wisely. Freedom, that irreducible category, can surpass conditioning sometimes.

In the terrible world system in which we live, optimism has become so degraded that it has nothing to do with happiness for Sartre—it is simply that we do not suffer for nothing. But in our world of almost entirely alienated *praxis*, we cannot even be sure of this. The writer who is outside the world, who feels he does not belong, the bastard, is in the best position to elucidate the human reality others seem so caught up in. The world is a prison without bars in which individual or collective realization is not now possible, but the stern Sisyphean Sartre can at least contest it.

# 2

# Schizoid Despair

Sartre's world-view is essentially a pessimistic one. The world is an unfriendly viscosity bereft of all meaning. Confronted with a godless world, man who is himself an absence has an abiding sense of futility. He is even denied control of the consequences of his action. A man is not what he wills himself to be—he is what he does.[1] Any immanent meaning can be discovered only after death. Sartre can even look at life from death backwards.[2] Loser so often wins.[3]

Paradoxes abound. Man is what he is not and is not what he is. As a void he seeks fulfilment which, in the nature of the case, is unattainable. Man seeks the absolute but is a "useless passion"! Human relations are intrinsically "locked in conflict" and sado-masochistic pleasures are poor substitutes for love and friendship. As the individual is an empty non-entity, life becomes a grim and constant

1. Sartre (1944), *In Camera*, p. 189.
2. Sartre, *Words*, pp. 125, 128.
3. While Sartre's focus has moved from the individual to the group, his under-lying framework does not alter greatly. *Altona* which is related to the *Critique de la raison dialectique* strikes the most sombre note in Sartre's work. The *Critique* itself is essentially pessimistic in its emphasis on violence and terror in and by the group. The possibility of a "third" emerging to save the situation can find no ground in the *Critique* itself. *Words*, which was first published in 1963, is a work of profound disillusion. Indeed, despite Sartre's occasional assertions that he is not describing the prevailing condition as a necessary one, no ground can be provided from within his framework such that the transcendence of it can count as a real possibility. Further, a number of readings of Sartre are possible. An exclusively explicit reading of Sartre will find many contradictions, while a solely implicit reading may reflect more of the reader than it does of Sartre. A balanced approach could take Sartre's own cue as a starting point in *What is Literature*? pp. 20-21 (partly quoted below).

struggle to preserve a minimal personal integrity against hostile others, or else a self-deceiving loss of identity in another person, ideology or organization. Man longs to escape the freedom to which he is condemned. But in this he is doomed to frustration and despair.

In a critique of *Being and Nothingness* Marcuse claims that Sartre's ontological categories are in fact historical ones.[4] They are a function of the kind of world men have fashioned for themselves through their practice over the centuries. The world described by Sartre is the alienated world of modern technological capitalism, and according to Marcuse it should be understood in these terms and not at a metaphysical face-value.

There can be little doubt that the contemporary world has many of the features Sartre describes. The success of his literary work is sufficient testimony to this—along with the pre-eminence of writers such as Kafka and Beckett. Many of the characters in modern literature lack what Laing terms "primary ontological security" in a way that those in earlier times did not.[5] Sartre's work vividly depicts the widespread problems of lack of personal identity, a sense of futility, feelings of impotence, and unfulfilling and hostile human relations. An analysis of Sartre's work may provide a clue to a deeper understanding of this world.

It is possible to divine an illuminating approach from Sartre himself in his discussions of his own work and in his criticism of that of others. Sartre is in fact a dialectical thinker in many ways: he turns back on himself, seeing what he has done from the standpoint of his having done it. He often "thinks against himself"[6] and attempts to understand the way he comes to the position he holds. Sartre's *Words*, an autobiography of his first ten years, is an attempt to comprehend the origins of his basic life structure. Sartre has upbraided Marxist theorists for ignoring the importance of childhood,[7] and himself believes that "childhood decides everything".[8]

Sartre has had a life-long obsession with Flaubert whom he sees as opposing everything he himself holds,[9] yet who bears so many similarities to Sartre that he may well represent Sartre's *alter ego*.[10] In his recent study of Flaubert Sartre's aim is "to try to determine

4. H. Marcuse, "Sartre's Existentialism" in his *Studies in Critical Philosophy*.
5. Laing, *The Divided Self*, Ch. 2.
6. Sartre, *Words*, p. 156. *See* also Sartre's "explanation" in "A Long Bitter-Sweet Madness", Encounter, XXII, p. 63.
7. Sartre, *Search for a Method*, p. 62.
8. Sartre, *Words*, p. 40.
9. Sartre, "A Long Bitter-Sweet Madness", p. 63.
10. F. Busi, "Sartre on Flaubert", *Research Studies* 41, pp. 14-16.

the encounter between the development of the person as psychoanalysis has shown it to us, and the development of history".[11] Perhaps Sartre was referring to his own past work when he wrote that:

> the dead from Montaigne to Rimbaud have portrayed themselves completely, but without having meant to. The surplus which they have given us unintentionally should be the primary and professed goal of all writers ... (S)ince we find pleasure in foiling the ruses of Chateaubriand and Rousseau, in surprising them in the secret places of their being at the moment they are playing at being the public man, in distinguishing their private motives from their most universal assertions, we shall ask newcomers to procure this pleasure deliberately. So let them reason, assert, deny, refute and prove: but the cause they are defending must be only the apparent aim of their discourse: the deeper goal is to yield themselves without seeming to do so ... Let them not presume to think in earnest: thought conceals the man and it is the man alone that interests us.[12]

In this light it is possible to explore Sartre's work to find not only the man but his world also. Such an understanding of Sartre's situation should provide illumination of the more general scene. Any sharp distinction between politics and individual psychology ignores how far the individual has internalized aspects of the macro-world, and how far the macro-world is constituted by micro-worlds. The individual person grows up in a number of contextual systems and interacts with them. As Sartre makes Franz say in *Altona*: "I am every man and all mankind. I am the century. Like anyone."[13] Or, as Sartre says of his autobiographical work, "through my story, it is that of my epoch that I want to transcribe".[14]

Marcuse claims that Sartre has mystified a historical situation. On a macro-level this is a function of a general alienation related to social structure (e.g. capitalist use of technology). An explanation of the manner in which the individual experiences and interacts with his world leads beyond conventional politics to encompass psychological phenomena.

The British object-relations school of psychoanalysis—in particular W.R.D. Fairbairn, D.W. Winnicott and Harry Guntrip—has gone far in providing a complete "psychological" account (as opposed to a psychobiological account of innate drives, affects, etc.) of personality structure which assumes that the child at birth is an

11. Sartre, "Itinerary of a Thought", p. 51.
12. Sartre, *What is Literature*? pp. 20-21.
13. Sartre, *Altona*, p. 126.
14. Sartre (1953), Interview, *Libération*. (My translation.)

energized pristine unitary ego (Fairbairn) which is object-seeking, and personality depends on his relationships with significant others particularly in the first years. Special interest is devoted to the events of the first six months of life in which the most basic ego-splits take place. Schizoid factors in the personality are the most deeply rooted, and very often the psychopathological processes which begin afterward serve as defences against them. According to Guntrip the schizoid problem concerns "people who have deep-seated doubts about the reality and validity of their very 'self', who are ultimately found to be suffering from various degrees of depersonalization, unreality, the dread feeling of 'not belonging', of being fundamentally isolated and out of touch with their world". These people "feel cut off, apart, different, unable to become involved in any real relationships".[15] Elsewhere he writes:

> (T)he schizoid sense of futility, disillusionment and underlying anxiety (is apparent) in existentialism. These thinkers, from Kierkegaard to Heidegger and Sartre, find human existence to be rooted in anxiety and insecurity, a fundamental dread that ultimately we have no certainties and the only thing we can affirm is "nothingness", "unreality", a final sense of triviality and meaninglessness. This surely is schizoid despair and loss of contact with the verities of emotional reality, rationalized into a philosophy. Yet existentialist thinkers, unlike the logical positivists, are calling us to face and deal with these real problems of the human situation. It is a mental sign of our age.[16]

The theme of *séquestration* (being locked up) provides a vital underlying theme in Sartre's work[17] In his literature the scenes are often set in rooms almost hermetically sealed off from the outer world. The room of the madman Pierre in "The Room", the second empire drawing room in *Huis Clos*, the room in *Morts sans sépulture* in which the resistance fighters await torture and death, Hoederer's room in *Les Mains sales* and that of Franz in *Altona* provide some examples. These symbolize man's situation as enveloped by forces beyond his control and in which he is condemned to a freedom it is impossible to use authentically, to an internal void that can never be filled, to human relations which are intrinsically frustrating and finally to death which destroys all significance. For Sartre, "Life does not only take place in a prison, it is in itself a prison".[18]

15. H. Guntrip, *Psychoanalytic Theory, Therapy and the Self*, p. 148.
16. H. Guntrip, *Schizoid Phenomena, Object-Relations and the Self*, p. 48. *See also* ibid., p. 290. The present discussion relates only to the work of Sartre. Whether what Guntrip says is true of, say, Heidegger is another question.
17. M.-D. Boros, *Un séquestre: l'homme sartrien*, p. 13.
18. S. Doubrovsky, "Sartre and Camus: A Study in Incarceration", *Yale French Studies* 25, p. 87.

Sartre's interest in *séquestration* finds its origin in his own childhood experience of being an only child without peers who was shut up in his grandfather's house where his only friends were his grandfather's books. Sartre's mother was treated as a child in the household which was ruled by Sartre's domineering grandfather. Sartre had no respect for her and came to regard his mother as an elder sister in need of his protection.[19] He was treated as a doll, a cute exhibition piece, an object—but never as a worthwhile person in his own right who had real and valid feelings of his own. The young Sartre's internal reality was systematically invalidated: his being became his being-for-others. Sartre felt his true self to be in the hands of the adults. Feeling empty, he was an impostor[20] playing the part he understood was expected of him by adults. The world of reason, books and ideas was substituted for the emotionally real, meaningful and confirming experience he lacked. He felt as malleable as clay, like a jellyfish inside[21] and was disgusted with what he saw as the "trivial unreality" of the world.[22]Sartre sees childhood as a "solitary" reality in which what the child internalizes is beyond his control.[23] It is scarcely surprising that his work denigrates the reality of feeling in favour of an intellectual rationality which sees man as a void, a lack, a nothingness.

Later, at university he felt cut off from the rest of the world: the suffering proletariat was only on the far horizon and the public world provided only a "backdrop" for his private life.[24] Sartre's first interest was literature—living life was quite subsidiary.[25]

Yet the world situation had consequences for all: Sartre's childhood experiences were confirmed in the larger historical situation. Especially from 1930 onward individual life "seemed governed down to the minutest details by obscure and collective forces, and its most private circumstances seemed to reflect the state of the whole world".[26] The individual could feel powerless, contingent, meaningless, cut off in an atomized, irrational, impersonal and Godless world. The individual's actions were stolen from him, seeming unrelated to his intentions or will. Having himself felt alienated and unreal since childhood, Sartre mistook the particular historical situation for the human condition as such.[27]

19. Sartre, *Words*, pp. 13-14.
20. Ibid., p. 53.
21. Ibid., p. 69.
22. Ibid., 143.
23. Sartre, *Search for a Method*, p. 18.
24. de Beauvoir, *The Prime of Life*, p. 57.
25. Ibid., p. 173.
26. Sartre, *What is Literature*?, p. 157.
27. Sartre, *Words*, p. 156.

During the war Sartre was imprisoned by the Germans in a camp in which he had his first experience of solidarity,[28] although then, and afterwards in the Resistance his role was not an active fighting one. Sartre's involvement through writing "often made me feel ashamed",[29] and he often wondered how he would react under torture.[30] In his own depersonalized state the world of those who actually fought, worked with their hands and had a cause seemed far more real than his own. This conformed to the prevalent Communist Party denigration of the intellectual as an inferior, a "useless mouth" who was involved with the Party not because of the harsh reality of circumstances, but because he became freely involved for principles such as justice and self-respect.[31]

In *Les Mains sales* Hugo, whose situation and childhood resemble Sartre's own, feels unreal, despicable, beyond help and untrusted. He joins the Party to forget himself and feel real and valuable through direct action. He hates everything and everybody, including himself, and cannot stop playing in a world in which he feels he has no place. He has no conviction of what is true and false, real and unreal. He does not know why he killed Hoederer and his only decisive and meaningful act is precisely the one which was to result in a meaningless death—his own. It is his only way out if he is to preserve his principles and purity. Not having a sense of inner value and security, he cannot accommodate to a situation where the principles which provide his *raison d'être* cannot meaningfully be employed in action. Sartre echoes the Stalinist conception that a man's intentions, however good they may be, are irrelevant: what matters are the objective consequences of actions. Thus Hoederer was an objective traitor who had to be eliminated. For Sartre, man is nothing: only what he does is relevant: "Doing reveals being."[32] Emotional reality is dissolved into an intellectual secondary discovery of the consequences of action. If a man has no internal personal reality, what he does is the only reality to which he can cling. If a man's being is his being-for-others revealed to him through what he does, then what others make of him is totally determining and potentially annihilating.

In human affairs Hoederer believed the good action to be the effective one—in politics one's hands are inevitably soiled. Those who opposed him in the Party were of his type, not Hugo's. Hugo greatly

28. de Beauvoir, *Force of Circumstance*, p. 13.
29. Sartre, *What is Literature?*, p. 173.
30. Ibid., p. 162.
31. Ibid., pp. 191-93.
32. Ibid., p. 175.

admires Hoederer, even wishing to assume his personality.[33] Hoederer is in a position to act pragmatically without recourse to abstract principles through which he can sustain himself. If Hugo's purity and principles become meaningless, he has nothing and is nothing. That is why death is the only way out. Sartre writes of the tragic paradox of our age in which "constructive freedom has never been so close to becoming conscious of itself and never has it been so profoundly alienated ... Never has *homo faber* better understood that he has *made* history and never has he felt so powerless before history".[34] Hugo has discovered this in his own version of "loser wins": the policies of Hoederer, the man he killed for the Party, have now become official Party policy.[35]

However there is another and deeper motive for Hugo's assassination of Hoederer. Hugo has no feeling of personal identity—indeed he sees himself as merely a reflection of his father.[36] Hugo joined the Party to enter a situation in which, contrary to his experience at home, there is truth rather than lies; in which he could be wanted and trusted for the first time in his life. He agrees to assassinate Hoederer so that he will derive a sense of inner value in being entrusted with an important mission.[37] When he becomes Hoederer's secretary, he finds in Hoederer his own ego-ideal. Hoederer tells Hugo he trusts him and will help him.[38] Although Hugo finds it difficult to trust another's trust in him since he does not trust himself, he goes to accept Hoederer's offer of help. Finding his wife in Hoederer's arms, Hugo says that he had suspected that Hoederer had ulterior motives in offering him his help. "I'm not angry with you (Jessica), and I'm not jealous either, we're not in love. But he, he very nearly caught me in his trap. 'I'll help you, I'll help you become a man.' What a fool I was! He didn't give a damn for me!"[39] The schizoid person, whose especially intense need of good relationship with another person is matched only by his fear of desertion and rejection by that same person, suspects all relationships for he has not had the confirmatory experience of basic trust in childhood.[40] With his defences down, Hugo was particularly vulnerable and found that his childhood experience was reconfirmed by the first person who could have

33. Sartre, *Crime Passionnel*, p. 107.
34. Sartre, *What is Literature?*, pp. 173-74.
35. Sartre, *Crime Passionnel*, p. 116.
36. Ibid., p. 24.
37. Ibid., p. 26.
38. Ibid., pp. 105-8.
39. Ibid., pp. 110-11.
40. Guntrip, *Schizoid Phenomena*, p. 220 ff. Guntrip, *Personality Structure*, p. 282 ff.

helped him replace it with a trusting and meaningful personal relationship.

*The Roads to Freedom* provides a self-portrait of Sartre during the pre-war and war years—for Mathieu Delarue is assuredly Sartre himself.[41] As the Hugo-Hoederer relationship is very important in *Les Mains sales*, so the Mathieu-Brunet relationship is vital in *The Roads to Freedom*. Mathieu, the indecisive, intellectualized, evasive, bourgeois, impotent, self-searching, empty philosophy teacher is counterposed to the solid, powerful, resolute, certain, real proletarian man of action, Brunet. Brunet, who looms so much larger than life for Mathieu, has a magical quality about him encompassing not only the room in which he sits, but the whole world of struggling masses.[42] Mathieu would like to be like Brunet but finds he cannot even reach first base. The reader witnesses Mathieu's loathesome and unreal existence which reaches its peak in his finding a meaning to his life by dying to demonstrate the impossibility of living, by his symbolic revenge for all his failures in life. His only definite, if putative, act is destructive. Mathieu is beset by paradox: in whichever direction he turns, there is no authentic exit.[43] He is imprisoned in the "unbarred cage"[44] he takes to be human existence. Duped by nature, man is, like Mathieu, nothing at all, or else he impersonates what he is, like Brunet.[45] Brunet achieves his calm certain solidity through being a soldier of the Party,[46] through renouncing his freedom in a type of religious conversion which brings him salvation.[47] Brunet, who seems a whole man, nothing but a man, is really a caricature of one. His very *raison d'être* is based on self-deception.

Thus Mathieu is ambivalent toward Brunet: he would love nothing more than to be like Brunet, but he could not achieve the leap of faith required without negating his own existence which places reason so far ahead of feeling.[48] By offering Mathieu the chance to join the Party, Brunet was offering him "the best thing in the world; everything would be rendered unto him".[49] But Mathieu cannot act without sufficient reason—conviction must follow reason, and not vice versa.[50]

41. Thody, *Sartre: A Biographical Introduction*, p. 84.
42. Sartre, *The Age of Reason*, pp. 116-20.
43. Sartre (1949), *Iron in the Soul*, pp. 203-25.
44. Sartre, *The Age of Reason*, p. 113.
45. Ibid., p. 173.
46. Ibid., p. 120.
47. Sartre, "Materialism and Revolution", p. 207.
48. Sartre, *The Age of Reason*, p. 42.
49. Ibid., pp. 118-21.
50. Ibid., p. 121.

For Mathieu there is a complete split between reason and feeling. A life based on reason alone is as much a lie as one based exclusively on feeling.[51] Mathieu buries himself ever deeper in the quagmire by his demand for absolute certainty. He sees himself as an embodied refusal whose identity would be at stake in a world in which he would have to say "Yes".[52] He defines himself *against*: he knows what he is by what he is not. His nothingness is that which distinguishes the boundary between himself and others, that which prevents his merging with them. Brunet is the Party—his words and actions belong to the Party. Brunet's strength and identity are dependent on a collusively accepted myth.

The alternatives open to Mathieu as he sees them are to lose his identity (renounce his freedom) by joining the Party, or to maintain his precarious identity by keeping his distance from the menacing world that threatens to overwhelm and engulf him. Mathieu has a constant grip on himself—feelings will never rule him. He will not let himself go for fear of losing himself. Feeling that there is nothing inside him is preferable to losing his inside altogether. To keep away from his feelings he represses them. His attachment to reason is rationalization. Refusing to confront his ambivalences, he cancels out opposing feelings in the defence of feeling just a nothingness. He feels that all he is is his shell.[53] Mathieu throughout neither explores nor experiences his core feelings—only those of his outer defences. His lack of commitment is not a happy one since there is nothing he desires more nor at the same time fears more. He can do neither with nor without relationship. If he forgets himself for a moment, flies and cockroaches appear. If he commits himself to an action, he will be robbed of its consequences—he will lose control.[54] Yet by not doing anything, he is pushed around by personal and impersonal forces which seem well beyond control. If he maintains his existence as stolid refusal, at least the refusal exists.

In spite of himself however, Mathieu has only a pseudo-independence. He feels so insecure that he relies on the outer world to give his life meaning. This characterizes the schizoid dilemma in which the self feels so empty that it relies on relationship with others precisely with whom it seems potentially suicidal to relate. Mathieu reaches a schizoid compromise in which he is "half-in and half-out" of relationship.[55] He is sympathetic to the Party but will not join, has

51. Guntrip, *Schizoid Phenomena*, p. 65.
52. Sartre, *The Age of Reason*, pp. 125, 299.
53. Sartre, *The Age of Reason*, pp. 186, 267, 300, 307-8.
54. Ibid., p. 299.
55. Guntrip, *Schizoid Phenomena*, p. 58 ff.

a lover but will not commit himself, rails at capitalism but remains an official, attacks bourgeois living while remaining a bourgeois ...[56] His compromise means diminished desires but also diminished rewards. Feeling is erased in his general state of continuous withdrawness.[57] He is never really unhappy, but his life is one of chronic frustration. He is free, but can never act. Mathieu is set in his ways—a static, rather predictable personality who is normally incapable of any but trivial acts of spontaneity.[58] He is cut adrift in his own futile world, floating aimlessly, waiting.[59] Yet he will run no risks: he is, as Ivich observes, too intelligent for that.[60] He sees too clearly, too straight, he understands and knows too much. In the aloofness and fastidiousness he so enjoys, Mathieu can remain cold, detached, even icy. Emotionally detached from others he is his own sternest critic in a life of continuous and gloomy introspection.[61] Even in his withdrawn state he sees himself as two: an analyst and analysand—the judging, critical analyst requiring full account from the analysand.

In finding a means of coping, Mathieu has committed a form of psychic suicide: devoid of feeling, how can he feel any point to life? Living becomes an intellectual exercise. In a life full only of missed opportunities Mathieu waits for a lightning flash which could fuse reason and emotion into a self-certain conviction.[62] This is precisely what his radically split ego cannot achieve. Mathieu sees himself as a rotter, a washout who needs to be thoroughly cleansed. All is libidinally bad within him. He hates himself and purification comes only in his putative suicide in which he takes revenge on his past failures through firing on the approaching Germans. This absurd and futile gesture renders him very potent and clean in his own eyes. His destructive feelings are acted out against the Germans as projections of himself. Killing his first German is his first definite action—it was *his* German. Formerly he had possessed nothing. Deliriously he wishes to plunge all Germany into mourning. Then he might have enough, perhaps even a self.

Mathieu, who had been living in a relatively stable schizoid state of withdrawness, had finally committed himself. What may be noted is the connection between commitment and destruction. He had

56. Sartre, *The Age of Reason*, pp. 106-7.
57. Guntrip, ibid., p. 64ff.
58. Sartre, *The Age of Reason*, p. 195, and *Iron in the Soul*, p.156.
59. Sartre, *The Reprieve*, p. 76, and *The Age of Reason*, p. 207.
60. Sartre, *The Age of Reason*, p. 73.
61. Ibid., pp. 13-14.
62. Ibid., p. 51. Sartre, *The Reprieve*, p. 308.

warned Pirette against taking up arms against the Germans, after which in spite of his better judgement, he took up a rifle in an action which could have none but a subjective meaning—he was holding up the German timetable by fifteen minutes. Although he realized he was dying for nothing, he saw that he was living for nothing, that life was meaningless to him. His commitment demonstrates the final loss of self on the one hand subjectively in a magical feeling of omnipotence, and on the other in reality actual self-annihilation. Commitment for Mathieu is life and death at the same time—doing what he most wants means self-annihilation.

For Sartre action means losing oneself in it. There is no autonomous self behind an action or role. The waiter sees himself and is seen primarily as a Waiter.[63] His role defines him—he cannot be *in* his actions without *being* his actions. For the schizoid the boundaries of the self may be those of his shell—being becomes the refusal to *be* anything. Commitment means engulfment. The self as shell remains by not being engulfed, for neither symbiosis nor aloneness is a viable alternative. Symbiosis means a total dependence on a constricting and frustrating mother who will contract to supply all needs only at the price of the child's soul. Aloneness is being cast out helpless without relationship into the unfriendly and untrustworthy menacing wilderness. Sartre's alternatives present an ego in the stage of infantile dependence, a state of identification with the parent.[64]

Sartre's analysis of being-for-others in *Being and Nothingness* confirms this. All human relationships are of a mutually devouring kind—one's being is swallowed up by another's and vice versa.

> While I attempt to free myself from the hold of the Other, the Other is trying to free himself from mine: while I seek to enslave the Other, the Other seeks to enslave me ... Conflict is the original meaning of being-for-others.[65]

All relationships involve either sadism or masochism—one attempts to "appropriate" the "freedom" of the Other or surrenders one's own to him. But "the Other is on principle inapprehensible; he flees me when I seek him and possesses me when I flee him".[66] Thus a satisfying sado-masochistic equilibrium is impossible—relationships are doomed to frustration. One wishes to "absorb" and "assimilate" the Other or be "absorbed" or "assimilated" by him. Being reliant

63. Sartre, *Being and Nothingness*, p. 101.
64. Guntrip, *Personality Structure*, pp. 391-92.
65. Sartre, *Being and Nothingness*, pp. 474-75.
66. Ibid., p. 529.

on the Other for recognition, one is in perpetual danger and has no security.[67] Apart from indifference—which is no relationship at all or withdrawal from relationship—hate is the only alternative relation to love. For Sartre hate involves my wishing the Other dead so that I will not be object for him.[68] The close relation of this hate to love is paralleled by Guntrip's view of hatred: it is

> love grown angry because of rejection. We can only really hate a person if we want their love. Hate is an expression of frustrated love needs, an attempt to destroy the bad rejecting side of a person in the hope of leaving their good responsive side available, a struggle to alter them.[69]

Sartre's picture of relationships is one which is proper to the first few months of life in the oral sucking attitude of the infant.[70] Feeling empty the frustrated and deprived infant feels a specially intense hunger to devour the breast so as to possess it entirely. Yet the anxiety created in the fear of exploiting the indispensable love object to the point of destruction may be so great as to lead to a withdrawal from all relationships which are seen as too dangerous to enter into.[71]

According to Sartre the self, as a nothingness, is so empty, so inherently deprived of satisfactory fulfilment that he feels he needs to be certain of the Other—which he cannot be by the nature of the Other's separateness and subjectivity. This leads to a sadistic drive to incorporate or absorb the Other with the concomitant fear of destroying the very person he desires. One wants to have the Other as subject or person, not as an object or instrument. But we cannot have our cake and eat it. One seeks to control and secure the freedom of the Other, but it is precisely the unconstrained freedom of the Other, upon which the self cannot depend, that is required for secure recognition.[72]

Sartre's conceptions of being-for-others in the outer world are generated by the emotions of the inner world. The relationships that Sartre describes reflect the internal bad objects of a barely developed inner world. The Other upon whom the self cannot rely is the breast that may be snatched away at any time. As Guntrip remarks, "The

67. Ibid., pp. 477-78.
68. Sartre, *Being and Nothingness*, pp. 532-34.
69. Guntrip, *Schizoid Phenomena*, p. 26.
70. Hate is related more to the subsequent oral biting stage of the second six months. Naturally this is related to the first period.
71. Guntrip, *Schizoid Phenomena*, p. 35.
72. Sartre, *Being and Nothingness*, p. 478 ff. It should be noted that Sartre's ontology is itself a schizoid one: the for-itself (which is already split from the body) is ineluctably split from the in-itself. Being and Nothingness are utterly irreducible categories and for Sartre human reality lacks being by definition.

schizoid is very sensitive and quickly feels unwanted, because he is always feeling deserted in his inner world".[73] Guntrip's description of the schizoid who cancels his object-relations because they are too frustrating, frightening and dangerous, applies to so many of Sartre's situations.

> Retreat into indifference is the true opposite of the love which is felt to be too dangerous to express. Want no one, make no demands, abolish all external relationships, and be aloof, cold and without any feeling, do not be moved by anything. The withdrawn libido is turned inwards, introverted. The patient goes into his shell and is busy only with internal objects towards who he feels the same devouring attitude. Outwardly and in consciousness everything seems futile and meaningless ... The depressive fears loss of his object. The schizoid, in addition, fears loss of his ego, of himself.[74]

*Huis Clos* is a dramatization of Sartre's analysis of being-for-others in *Being and Nothingness*.[75] The three occupants constantly thwart and frustrate each other in the hermetically closed second empire drawing-room which is their Hell. Garcin concludes that "Hell is other people",[76] for each person acts as torturer to the other two. However, at one stage the door to their prison opens to Garcin's insistant knocking, but no one, including Garcin, leaves. They are "inseparables". Garcin claims that his reason for not leaving and for his not pushing Inez—who hates him—out of the room is his need for her confirmation.[77] However, if Hell really is other people, why does no one leave?

*Huis Clos* may be regarded as an image of the inner bad object world which is a "closed system" that is a "static internal situation".[78] This closed system is what Sartre's concern with *séquestration*, with imprisonment, is basically about. This inner world of bad objects, revealed by Melanie Klein, is understood by Fairbairn to constitute "the most formidable resistance in psychoanalytical treatment".[79] This inner world is often dreamed of as a torture house, a prison or a concentration camp in which the self is a prisoner.[80] This system is "run on hate", and the self is the victim of a large amount of persecution. Of course the prison in

73. Guntrip, *Schizoid Phenomena*, p. 28.
74. Ibid., p. 27.
75. Sartre, *Being and Nothingness*, Part Three, Ch. 3.
76. Sartre, *In Camera*, p. 191.
77. Sartre, *In Camera*, pp. 187-88.
78. W.R.D. Fairbairn, "On the Nature and Aims of Psychoanalytical Treatment", *International Journal of Psychoanalysis* 39, p. 38.
79. Ibid., p. 38.
80. Guntrip, *Schizoid Phenomena*, p. 198ff.

which the person finds himself has been erected by himself. But it is a prison which it is very difficult to breach, and this indicates just how strongly the person holds on to his persecutory system of internal object-relations. Many people do not want to leave their prisons—it is far more dangerous outside.[81]

The persecutory internal object-relationship is that of the internalized bad parents whom it is impossible to do without, since the person would then be all alone without any relationship at all. It is better to be hated than ignored—far better be something than nothing. The closed system is part of a struggle to keep going, to have some degree of independence. Further, the internal closed system of persecution "confers a sense of power, if only over the self".[82] Identification with powerful objects, even where these are self-destructive, gives some security. Guntrip writes:

> The entire world of internal bad objects is a colossal defence against loss of the ego by depersonalization. The one issue that is much worse than the choice between good and bad objects is the choice between any sort of objects and no objects at all. Persecution is preferable to depersonalization.[83]

This is why the imnates in *Huis Clos* dare not leave their prison. Garcin, for example, has a hate relationship with Inez, which is preferable to being alone in absolute isolation. Further, since Estelle is of no account to Garcin, it is imperative that Inez stay to provide a meaningful, if hostile, relationship. The worst ultimate terror is to be a "psyche in a vacuum".[84] The irresolvable relationships of *Huis Clos* are staunch defences against personal annihilation. Hell is not other people—it is being utterly alone.

This is very clear in one of Sartre's first stories, "Erostratus".[85] The ancient Greek, Erostratus, achieved notoriety by burning down the temple of Diana at Ephesus. Nobody remembers the builder of the temple, but its destroyer became immortal. In Sartre's story Hilbert carries out Breton's pure surrealist act:[86] he takes a rifle and shoots randomly at people in the street. Instantly this nobody became recognized as somebody. It is better to be a "bad somebody" than a "weak nonentity".[87]

81. Guntrip, *Personality Structure*, p. 422.
82. Guntrip, *Schizoid Phenomena*, p. 205.
83. Guntrip, *Personality Structure*, pp. 431-32.
84. Guntrip, *Schizoid Phenomena*, p. 238.
85. Sartre, "Erostratus".
86. Sartre, *What is Literature*?, p. 99.
87. Guntrip, *Schizoid Phenomena*, p. 137.

Futility is a basic theme in *Nausea* which chronicles a period of the existence of Roquentin.[88] Roquentin is overwhelmed by the viscous, elusive, non-graspable character of being itself.[89] He experiences himself as a dull and jelly-like sensation, and is a constant observer of his own lack of involvement in an essentially meaningless world. Self-conscious, Roquentin keeps constant watch over himself for fear that he may disappear. He has no place in the world and feels no sense of continuity. Alone in a crowd, a stranger everywhere, he is essentially cut off from any sense of reality.[90] Life is a constant struggle to preserve a precarious individuation as any sort of ego at all. All resources are employed to maintain this separation. The nothingness Roquentin experiences as himself is a defence against engulfment or impingement by an overwhelming reality.[91] The ego is withdrawn into the deepest recesses of the self, out of reach of being hurt, while at the same time, a wall is erected around himself keeping reality at a distance. Thus alienated it would be impossible to feel anything but futile. For security is a function of good object-relations.[92] A feeling of inner value and integrity can only emerge from a warm, reliable human relationship that is personal on both sides through which growth toward autonomy in relationships of mature dependence may occur. The beginnings of autonomy should emerge in the first six months of life.

This schizoid world of Sartre's need not be viewed solely through the eyes of the British object-relations school. The close relation the schizoid problem bears to narcissistic disorders[93] would make a study of Sartre's world in terms of the concept of narcissism well worthwhile. Further, the work of Erikson throws much light on many of Sartre's categories—especially through Erikson's development of the "eight stages of man" from basic trust and mistrust through to ego integrity. Each of these stages represents a radical change in perspective, an epigenesis, and an exploration of Sartre's work using Erikson's categories would show how Sartre's world is based mainly around the first psycho-social stage of "basic trust v. basic mistrust", and to a lesser extent involves the second, "autonomy v. shame

88. Sartre writes in *Words*: "I *was* Roquentin ... Mystified and a fraud to my very bones, I cheerfully wrote about out wretched lot". (p.156) Yet the reader of *Words* does not find an essentially different Sartre from the writer of *Nausea*, Sartre is as disillusioned as ever.f
89. *See also* Sartre, *Being and Nothingness*, Part Four, Ch. 2.f
90. Sartre, *Nausea*, p. 191 ff.f
91. Ibid., p. 181.f
92. Guntrip, *Schizoid Phenomena*, p. 238.f
93. Ibid., pp. 42-43.

and doubt".[94] In any case many other themes in Sartre's work (e.g. treachery, giving and receiving, dependence, embodiment) could be usefully looked at in detail in terms of psychologies of the oral stage of development.

Sartre's world is certainly one of schizoid despair (though not entirely so as we shall see in the following chapter). But it is not his individual problem alone—Sartre is a man of this age. The problems raised are among the most pervasive and profound of this era. They invite the question: How is the prevailing schizoid despair to be overcome so that most people may become "ontologically secure"?

94. E. Erikson; *Childhood and Society*, Ch. 7, and "Identity and the Life Cycle", *Psychological Issues* I, Ch. 3.

# 3

# Words and Reality

In this chapter I shall attempt to come to terms with the tension in Sartre's work between words and reality which seem worlds apart. The world of writing and the imaginary stand in stark relief against the world which is actually described in Sartre's literature, and the context in which Sartre himself overcomes the vision of reality depicted in his writing can be understood through the world of writing, of art itself. The ambivalence he has towards words and their relation to reality will be shown and his attitude may be seen as a way of coping with the ambiguities of reality, writing and action.

Sartre's work can be understood in terms of a number of frames of reference. This chapter will focus on the axes of writing and creativity and their relation to his ironic vision of reality. For ambiguity, paradox, absurdity and their inherent ironies define a reality in which what we want most—the absolute—is precisely that which we cannot attain, and we are all too aware of this. Sartre writes of his "missed vocation" as a priest, but the absence of God is displaced by devotion to the world of literature. If God would no longer assure immortality, literature could do so. Time and again Sartre has described himself as a Writer, and describes the duties thereof.[1] He is not a man who writes, is involved in politics, love, etc., but primarily a Writer. If literature isn't everything, it is nothing.[2] Literature is not integrated into life, but literature is a weapon to transform life itself: *What is Literature*? is a work of messianic zeal. Sartre even compares his literary mission with the religious,[3] and the communists who appear in his work derive their strength and identity from the

1. For example in Sartre, *What is Literature*? and in "To show, to Demonstrate", pp. 42-44.
2. Sartre, "To Show, To Demonstrate", p. 30.
3. Ibid., pp. 39-41, "Forgers of Myths", p. 332, and in *Words*, p. 39.

Party as the soldiers of Christ are nourished by the Holy Trinity.

His autobiography is entitled *Words*, and consists of two sections: "Reading" and "Writing". He tells there of the fascinating world to be found in his grandfather's library which stood in stark contrast to the dreary world of his bourgeois family and their friends. The "real" world was nowhere as alive as that of literature. Sartre's reality in his formative years was the fantasy world of literature, and the external world was an unfortunate diversion, the demands of which he satisfied by acting the model boy. From then on literature provided the centre of his life-project. *Words* traced back to his original choice to write, as Sartre's biographies of Baudelaire, Genet and Flaubert illuminate the conditions of their original choice to write. Once this choice has been disclosed everything thereafter becomes clear, as in a "life-script". Literature is a sword or it is impotent.[4] Sartre latterly discovers that what he saw as the sword to slash through mystifications and bring about a new era has failed—all or nothing. Sartre has staked his life on the word and until recently wrote voluminously, not through force of habit but, at least partly, because his life has been invested in it.[5]

Spontaneous political maoist activism today has been mixed with the most immense work in the imaginary that he has written—*L'Idiot de la famille*. His obsession with Flaubert almost exclusively consumed his literary efforts over the past number of years that the second volume of the *Critique*, not to mention a sequel to *Words*, were not written. His inexhaustible literary energy produced exhausting tomes, while much of the remainder of his existence has been spent in direct politics. He has been living in two worlds now radically split apart from each other. "In the beginning was the Word" and the Word has been absorbed and rendered powerless in a world in which God now seems well and truly dead. The resigned inner phantasy world remains however, and "never a day without a line"[6] has been the motto of a man who now sees literature as impotent in the world of men. Sartre's "missed vocation" may well have been one that had not so surely been missed as his vocation seems to Sartre to have done. In any case God's absence provides a major theme in Sartre's work with words.

Sartre is pre-eminently a man of words. The mysterious, magical world of words which so intoxicates Sartre seems to achieve an

4. Sartre, *Words*, p. 157, and "To Show, To Demonstrate", p. 44.
5. "To Show, To Demonstrate", p. 44, and interview with Contat, *Le Nouvel Observateur*.
6. Sartre, *Words*, p. 157, and "To Show, To Demonstrate", p. 36.

autonomous existence. At their best words will act as mirror to a reality through which men will see their condition and change the world in accordance with their ideals. To name something is to change it.[7]

Yet all along—and especially after the second world war—Sartre has been aware of the powerlessness and uselessness of words in contrast to action. Just as in childhood he envied other children their games while he stood on the sidelines,[8] as under the Occupation he felt guilty about not having an active fighting role in which he risked everything,[9] so he envies those who work with their hands, join the Party out of hardship, and are engaged in concrete action. As an intellectual he had no place in the Party of the working class, but as a radical there was no place in the comfortable world of the bourgeoisie either. Caught between two worlds, Sartre can see both from the edges—although the major part of his work is concerned with the world of the bourgeoisie. He became involved with the "third world" countries only in the later part of his life. Metaphysics takes second place in a world in which there are so many people without enough to eat.[10] His admiration for China, Cuba, and the newly emerging states in Africa, South America and Asia may remind us of his guilt about being a bourgeois intellectual who merely writes and does not work with his hands; is involved with the Party out of choice and not out of need; leaves the "real" fighting and risks to the soldiers of the cause who actually plant the bombs, assassinate leaders, or print underground literature. This is by no means to detract from Sartre's very real political courage: it is simply to point to the nagging and largely unrealistic guilt and, at the same time, envy of those who come face to face with dangers and privations which are necessities of their condition and potential liberation.

It should be added that the landscapes of contemporary western society painted in Sartre's work point to the absorption of the working class—Marx's historical vehicle of revolution—in western capitalist countries together with the virtual reformism and assimilation of communist parties there (in particular the Parti Communiste Francais although he had a good deal of sympathy with the Italian C.P.[11]) and the solidification of repression in the bureaucratic-technocratic communist countries. In these countries, the hope of a

7. Sartre (1947), "The World as Mirror", *Saturday Review of Literature*. XXX.
8. Sartre, *Words*, p. 84.
9. Sartre, *What is Literature*?, p. 173.
10. Sartre, "A Long Bitter-Sweet Madness", p. 62. Sartre (1964) "Sartre and the Nobel Prize", *New York Review of Books*. I
11. Contat and Rybalka, p. 401.

"third" emerging to save them seems remote—and it seems only in the "third" world that hope may lie for salvation. Yet it is precisely in these countries that Sartre's profession of words stands in greatest relief against the actual militant action needed to overcome oppression. Sartre's latest maoism may be seen in this light. So too can his literature of extreme situations—situations in which talking under torture matters, the word "No" has meaning and may mean death.

Words too may separate us from involvement and commitment. One word, laments Mathieu, and the real world of the Party could have been his.[12] Hugo cannot kill Hoederer because, as Hoederer says, an intellectual always has to think, and there are always reservations about any action.[13]

Sartre manifests an ambivalent attitude towards words and the world of writing—one which is manifested in the separation of politics and writing as much as in his conviction that the writer must be committed. This call to commitment reflects a reality—both internal and external—in which there is a very strong tendency in the opposite direction. The greater the messianic zeal Sartre exhibits in regard to the influence of literature, the greater is the problem revealed about the impotence of words. The world of the man of words, even in the forties is for Sartre one which is a world apart. His own philosophical writings, fiction and plays of the period do not seem to manifest the qualities of the *engagement* of *What is Literature*? Certainly they show the problems very clearly indeed, but this is quite a different matter. The intellectual sees himself as an individual who does not want to lose his identity in submergence in an organization. There is, of course, good reason for doing so when he does not have enough to eat, is the subject of direct physical aggression by the state and so on; but there does not seem to be this excuse in the advanced countries. The metaphysical problems which may be shelved in the third world are prominent in the first. Sartre's remonstrances that he is not a communist, can be taken to indicate "the existential problem of *becoming* a communist". For the C.P. is not a community that can overcome individual alienation by reconciling "the condition of reflection and action".[14]

His largest directly political work, *The Communists and Peace*, was written compulsively—he would write or suffocate.[15] This is a special instance of the function of words for Sartre: they are

12. Sartre, *The Age of Reason*, p. 124.f
13. Sartre, *Crime Passionnel*, p. 104.f
14. Cumming, "The Literature of Extreme Situations", p. 40.f
15. Sartre, "Merleau-Ponty", pp. 287-88. de Beauvoir, *Force of Circumstance*, p. 274.

both powerful and powerless. Words often pour out and flow easily—too easily. They come in a torrent which need never end. The intoxication with words can be seen in Sartre's virtual neglect of footnoting exactitude, or even accurate quotation.

Sartre seems to become enthralled in his own productions, and becomes the vehicle for the "automatic writing" machine:[16] he is absorbed in the world of words. *Saint Genet* emerged from a mere preface, and his work on Flaubert takes on an immense momentum of its own, for Sartre is the instrument of his language.

But the word captures the image more clearly than the image itself can directly show.[17] The world of words seems to become one approaching direct action, yet Sartre also knows it is not. Hamlet's "Words! Words! Words!" finds a modern incarnation in Hugo who feels unreal in a life which seems all words and no action, but in which he cannot act. Better be a good journalist than a bad assassin, Hoederer tells Hugo,[18] but the intellectual is free—free for nothing. He is too far from the realities of life, and does not have a home in the Party. He does not belong there and is a bastard. He uses words for want of action,[19] and must continuously earn his status of stepchild in the Party (Sartre describes his arguments with the Party as a "family quarrel" or affair).

The constant flow of words that seem unreflective does not often describe a living reality—or rather describes a reality in which the living seem dead. Rationalizations, strange and mysterious turns of phrase in Sartre's private vocabulary surge outward, mainly in his non-fictional and non-dramatic work. Sartre rarely discounts earlier work or comments, but often tries to explain how he has been "misunderstood". A dialectical turn of phrase attempts to capture the evasive human reality, and may convince Sartre for an instant that he has done so. At his best he does, but Sartre however is often anything but precise. An undifferentiated flow of words circles its object, touching it only at times. The words are dense or vague, perceptive or deceptive, meaningful or irrelevant ... in any case they seem to inhabit a world of their own.

The early Sartre sees transcendence of the abysmal human condition through art—as well as through the commitment of the writer. Words must move mountains, they must unmask and demystify meanings for the writer has a mission. The intellectual makes an important place for himself; yet this place, however acclaimed or effec-

16. Sartre, "The Word as Mirror"
17. Sartre, *Saint Genet*, p. 455 ff.
18. Sartre, *Crime Passionnel*, p. 107.
19. Sartre, *What is Literature*?, pp. 191-92.

tive, is only provisional even at its best. His reality is stolen from him by the mere fact of his bourgeois birth. Revolution becomes *engagement*, the making of reality. He can participate on the side of the proletariat, justice and can justify terror for the cause. Words are malleable and can justify anything. They are inherently powerful for this reason, but for this reason also they have no independent reality. The world of words alone is unreal—the mind can dream anything and there seem to be no definite consequences. Language can mutilate and deform through its communication too—how can we ever be sure that words reflect the world?

Sartre's characterizations so often skirt around the subjects—not revealing their inner selves, perhaps because there do not seem to be any. The characters generally seem less than men, and tragedy is not normally appropriate where the characters themselves are so detached that they are sometimes even unsure whether events take place at all. Hugo wonders who fired the revolver, or whether it fired at all. Did anything happen or was it a dream?[20] We can be as unsure as the small Genet whether what we take to be illusion is reality or vice versa, whether our reality is their reality or what they want us to believe. In any case the intellectual and the bastard feel unreal in the "real" world to which they do not belong.

Sartre becomes caught up in the self-enclosed world of ideas and words: outer reality becomes irrelevant, derealized and illusory. The magic power of words might transform it. But on the other hand it is powerless in actual confrontation with it—all and nothing. "For whom does one write?" and "What is writing?" are fundamental questions for Sartre as they reflect the omnipotence of writing in *phantasy*, and at the same time the impotence in the face of action in *reality*. Both are true for the committed messianic writer as the pen as sword can be seen as a point of contact with the world it so defiantly reveals. Words are a universal medium mediating and simultaneously mediated by the social totality. Thus in an era in which the social whole has entered and often nearly swamped the individual, words must be understood in their role, not only as potential liberators or demystifiers, but, on the contrary, as adding to and perpetuating prevailing ideologies.

Sartre, who holds Flaubert and the Goncourts responsible for the repression following the Paris Commune because they did not speak against it,[21] himself now sees literature as of no social import. People can read his work as they eat a piece of pie; they may read a book

20. Sartre, *Crime Passionnel*, p. 16.
21. Sartre, "The Case for Responsible Literature", p. 307.

without being its readers.[22] Sartre is aware that especially in the post-war world we use a language that is too old for us; words have become detached from their objects and seem to assume a reality of their own, just as many acts now seem to be without authors any more. The words are cut adrift and people may have the feeling that their language does not quite belong to them.[23] Words are social, they universalize[24] and at the same time express our condition. The literature of a period is that period pondered by literature.[25]

Sartre's ambivalence toward literature then reflects the way he sees his time, or perhaps his way of living his time. If literature can show, unveil, demonstrate, then it is what men do with this literature that matters.[26] Men have done nothing with it in the sense that they have not changed the world—or even France—using Sartre's visions. Sartre's concern with not being an institution[27] constitutes the awareness that writing is only one step in communication. Our words do not remain our own when they enter the market, and besides, every reader reads himself into the book.

Literature for Sartre had constituted salvation, a form of immortality which he no longer accepts.[28] He believes everyone should write to keep the forces of the night at bay.[29] In the case of Genet, writing constituted his liberation, but more recently Sartre sees Genet's liberation as having ended. His liberation lay in his writings which reflected his struggle against prison life and humiliation. "The fact of being 'Genet the Poet' led to a presidential pardon for 'Genet the Criminal'—but also to the drying up of the source of his poetry."[30]

Can this be true in the case of Sartre himself? *Words* marks his cure from the myths of literature. Since its publication only his diffuse biographical work on Flaubert has appeared—not any plays or fiction. Certainly it must be conceded that the Flaubert work attempts a most important task, but why had he written nothing else? Formerly he had used the pen as a sword, and now realizes how useless we are.[31] Changing the world will not occur through the medium of literature, but through action. Literature would not bring

22. Sartre, "To Show, To Demonstrate", p. 36.
23. Sartre, *Saint Genet*, p. 276.
24. Ibid., p. 436.
25. Sartre, "To Show, To Demonstrate", p. 30.
26. Ibid., p. 42.
27. Sartre, "Sartre and the Prize".
28. Sartre, "To Show, To Demonstrate", p. 40.
29. Ibid., p. 44.
30. Sartre, *Playboy* Interview, p. 168.
31. Sartre, *Words*, p. 157.

salvation, and writing came to seem more of a need, an emotional investment.[32]

In any case, Sartre has maintained the firm distinction between the worlds of politics and writing. It is worth quoting an example. In an interview with *Le Monde* he states:

> And before all else I'd like to tell you that I am a writer; that I have never gone in for politics, and never will, in the sense of "making a profession" of politics ... I am incompetent on the level of technical political action. Politics, in so far as it concerns me, is limited to the use I make of my ballot. If what I write reflects the miseries of our age and the way out of them which I glimpse, it is as a writer that I deal with them and I'm glad of it.[33]

Sartre was until recently involved with the production of a revolutionary newspaper, does not use his ballot and believes in illegality. As a writer he has tried to understand how we can know a man—Flaubert—the implications of which go well beyond the nineteenth century.[34] Thus while related ultimately with the human condition, literature and politics remain quite different and relatively autonomous worlds. The emphasis seems however to have shifted, literature now taking a second place to politics. The cure of his illusions described in *Words* meant that Sartre had become "a member of society",[35] or at least partly. Sartre's disillusionment with the salvific nature of literature has become compensated for to a degree by his involvement in a politics of voluntarism and spontaneity. Ten years ago he would not have believed a revolution to be possible, but now it "appears probable". However even if this were to occur in France, it would probably be crushed from outside.[36] Here we find again the problem of self and other in *Being and Nothingness*: the Other may crush my freedom. Sartre may well have found in politics today and in his interest in youth some of what he found in solidarity in the last world war and what he missed in not having played games with others in his own childhood. His "membership of society" contains however the old sense of Sisyphean defiance that informs most of his work, not the Promethean vision of an open future.

Sartre has enacted a version of the final conversion of Goetz from a struggle for God's recognition to a resigned and contradictory

32. Sartre, "To Show, To Demonstrate", p. 44.
33. Sartre, "... Said Jean-Paul Sartre", p. 5.
34. Sartre (1973), "On Maoism: an Interview with Jean-Paul Sartre", *Telos*, 16 pp. 99-101.
35. Sartre, *Playboy* Interview,p. 176.
36. Sartre, "On Maoism", p. 97.

struggle for mankind's liberation in the absence of God. Literature would no longer confer any immortality or salvation—perhaps political activity can have some meaning in the absence of the power of literature, especially where a concrete "third" may enter in the form of the "third world" struggles and ideologies—particularly maoism.

But as has been argued so far, Sartre's problematic is Sisyphean rather than Promethean, closed rather than open, schizoid rather than integrated. Even were the socio-economic ills of the world to be alleviated, our profound metaphysical position would remain the same and become clear to everyone. And literature itself can be seen as a false god since it could not constitute but at most reflect the world.

Perhaps the messianic role of Sartre's ideal of committed literature was a reaction to the content and direction of the world of Sartre's actual literature. The meaningless, futile and despairing world in which the consequences and meaning of action were stolen from actors who were nothing but their actions, and in which there was no escape hatch, no way out, somehow magically co-existed with a doctrine of salvation through *engagement*. How is this apparently glaring contradiction to be comprehended? We turn to some psychoanalytic explanations and then pursue the themes of play, and ironic play and vision in order to attempt such an understanding.

Traditional Freudian interpretation has concentrated on the release of tension and the sublimative aspects of writing.[37] Further analytic writers elucidated the narcissistic and exhibitionistic impulses motivating art work.[38] Bergler in a most revealing piece[39] found the basic role played by orality in writing. The writer manifests a spiteful desire for oral independence in identifying with the "giving" mother in writing, and eliminates her out of aggression towards her. The writer establishes an autarchic pseudo-independence by refuting the bad pre-oedipal mother together with the disappointments experienced through her. Oedipal conflicts often serve as defences against more basic oral conflicts.[40] The writer overcomes the disappointments of childhood by the equation of milk and the beautiful ideas and words which flow from the writer's pen.[41]

37. S. Freud, "The Relation of the Poet to Daydreaming" in *Character and Culture*.
38. A. Storr, *The Dynamics of Creation*, Ch. 1.
39. E. Bergler, "Psychoanalysis of Writers and of Literary Productivity", *Psychoanalysis and the Social Sciences*. I.
40. Ibid., pp. 250-51.
41. Ibid., p. 283.

The writer becomes not only the giving mother but the receiving child at the same time as the writer, among other things, is giving himself the words. The writer resolves his conflicts through writing.[42]

Bergler's explanation is however a reductionist one and does not explain the dynamic content nor quality of the artist's work. But his emphasis on the oral narcissistic quality in writers is valuable. Without reducing art to neuroses, Storr emphasizes creativity as a defence against anxiety. The schizoid person feels he has no place in the human hierarchy since at a very early age he has ceased to interact with his peers. He becomes preoccupied with inner rather than outer reality, and seeks meaning in systems rather than through human relations. Because what happens seems to the child to have no relation to his feelings, the world will appear to be ruled by capricious giants in an entirely arbitrary manner. The artist may show himself and his vision through his art and enjoy the gratifications of self-revelation, while being protected by the very medium of communication. He can communicate without being found. Creativity allows the phantasy of omnipotence, and some form of order can be imposed on the chaos that seems to exist in the outer world without the artist's being involved in relationships which seem to be full of danger.

Much of this applies to Sartre. He was never treated as a person in his own right and he experienced himself as a void. He discovered the world of the imaginary in his grandfather's library in which the world lay "trapped in a mirror",[43] wrote "novels" at an early age, and one day, while talking about his future with his grandfather, decided to become a writer. His ambition was to become a professor of literature like his grandfather, and he studied philosophy in order to enter the Ecole Normale Superieure.[44] Literature was his first and constant love, and Sartre has always identified himself as a writer. Sartre notes in *Words* that it had been pointed out to him that he acted as if he had no childhood,[45] and he feels that he had no identity with the person who "bore his name" at any previous time.[46] He refuses to admit any relation with his body and in the same way, de Beauvoir wrote in 1946 in similar vein:

> Sartre refuses to admit any identity with his past life. He seldom indulges

42. Ibid., p. 289.
43. Sartre, *Words*, p. 33.
44. Sartre, *Playboy* Interview, p. 167.
45. Sartre, *Words*, p. 148.
46. Ibid., p. 149.

> in reminiscences; he admits his mistakes with disconcerting candour; he can describe and criticise himself with strict impartiality. The truth is that he has already ceased to recognize himself in the former Sartre of whom he speaks ... His real likeness, he thinks, exists in the future, and hence he never feels any vanity about what he has done in the past.

He is one with his activity, accepting a liberty which tries to be absolute and refuses to be chained by circumstances. "He expects nothing from others but everything from himself." Further "He feels that nausea or revulsion in the face of everything contingent and tasteless, and, on the other hand, joy at surmounting the 'given' and existing as liberty, are the two phases of a single experience".[47]

Sartre then is described as pure activity, without a past or any continuous existence. What he expects from himself is this constant flow, and from the world nausea or tastelessness. A psychoanalytic interpretation is obvious, especially in view of his childhood experiences, and even in the light of his philosophy which postulates a radical split between the *pour-soi* which is the ceaseless activity of a nothingness which can never *be* anything, and the *en-soi* which is full of being; a massive, inert, repulsive and nauseating "mother" nature. No rapprochement is possible, and Sartre, who is a never ceasing activity, gives himself the milk deprived him by a mother whose milk is tasteless or nauseating, and from whom nothing whatever may be expected. The literature which is salvation is the milk of paradise which Sartre may dispense and enjoy in a feeling of basic independence.

The world of literature provides a counterpoint to the environment it depicts. Indeed Sartre's literature, which is so full of oral imagery, is pure and clean as opposed to the world of politics, for example, which is dirty, paradoxical and beyond one's control.

Of course Sartre would not accept a psychoanalytical explanation as more than an important aid to discovering how we may know a man, for we must always reckon with man's ineluctable and irreducible freedom. Praxis can never be reduced to process, even where it appears to be such. Nevertheless, psychoanalytical explanation can illuminate the setting, but it cannot properly explain it. There is always the person Sartre who refuses any attempt to reduce him out of existence. Certainly writing may have acted as a defence against a fundamental acceptance of futility. But it is precisely the nature and dynamic of that creativity, the exercise of that freedom which will now be explored.

The two aspects of Sartre's writing, resignation and despair with no possibility of redemption in the content, and literature as

47. de Beauvoir, "Jean-Paul Sartre: Strictly Personal", p. 160.

therapeutic, as salvation, as the method, will be understood on another level in terms of a third category: freedom. Sartre remarks that Genet's ten years of writing amounted to a "psychoanalytical cure",[48] and that this "cure" was to be understood ultimately in terms of freedom. Further he sees Genet the celebrated poet as having dried up, and feeling alone. Sartre himself gave that impression of himself strongly in *Words*, and his politics now seem to have taken a less lonely path. I shall now pursue an understanding of this in the case of Sartre through the category of play.

The rôle of play and games in Sartre's life and work is important. The child Sartre felt he was nothing, but played at being the model child. The Waiter plays at being the role ascribed to him and which he ascribes to himself. Lucien Fleurier plays at being an anti-semite. Brunet plays the Party man and Hugo cannot stop playing. Roquentin watches the eternal card games in the café, the games of the lovers at the adjacent table, and the games of the *salauds* promenading on a Sunday. Goetz wagers with God—and cheats—while everybody in *Altona* plays loser wins. The girl on a date tries not to notice her companion's sexual intents and scarcely recognizes her hand when it slips into his. The humanists play at loving Humanity, but only love the abstract Man; and the child Genet plays at being the Thief that society tells him he is. Kean the man does not know when he is Kean the actor, and vice versa. There seems no way of distinguishing reality and reflection in the hall of mirrors which so often turns out to be ultimately empty.

> Kean is Genet, Goetz, Hugo. More exactly, he is their perfect *representation*. "He is the very Myth of the Actor," said Sartre. "The actor who never stops playing, who plays his very life without recognizing it any more, without knowing who he is any longer. And who, in the end, is nobody." This Myth, by the same logic, then finds itself to be that of the Intellectual-bastard, traitor and actor all in one: the *Impostor, par excellence*.[49]

The impostor can only play at being, and the *esprit de sérieux* which might seem to justify a rôle is itself playing at justification. Play is ontologically necessary to Sartrean man who is by condition dual, consisting of reflexive and non-reflexive consciousness. We constantly play hide and seek with ourselves, always just eluding being hidden and being found.

If we cannot avoid playing, the articulate intellectual who is on the sidelines of the game is all too conscious of this. *Words* which finally

48. Sartre, *Saint Genet*, p. 544.
49. Jeanson, *Sartre par lui-même*, p. 75. (My translation).

brings the circumstances of the past to bear on Sartre himself is a piece of playful artistry, perhaps Sartre at his ironic and sardonic best. It is a work which is as delightful as it is resigned. The imaginary, which has fascinated Sartre since childhood, remains. "I began my life as I shall no doubt end it—among books."[50] It is the world of fantasy to which he can cheerfully take refuge. He dreams of living in a cell so as to be able to write in peace. He feels he is in a sixth floor room no matter where he is.[51] The free-floating fantasy world Sartre found in his grandfather's library was far preferable to the outside world. Sartre although deprived of peers found his friends among books, and events in the inner world took precedence over those of the external world. His playfulness is not together with others (except perhaps lately in politics), but in his own inner world. Given this situation, it is possible to understand how Sartre can be so cynical about the world and at the same time see something sacrosanct in literature. The outer world of his childhood could never achieve the dimensions the fantasy world of the library could offer.

Throughout his life Sartre is aware of the demands of the outer world and its impingement. Naturally his inner world is not simply that of his grandfather's library; it consists of a great variety of internalizations which occurred since birth. Thus the despair of his inner world finds its origins in the lack of recognition he received as a person in his own right, and the need for this recognition to allow any autonomy to develop. The joy and spontaneity of play with peers which was also denied him would have led him into despairing conformity, or more likely anomie (which is simply the reverse side of conformity) had he not found a refuge in the library. Play with others is impossible for Sartre, since he finds even authentic co-existence very difficult and dangerous. His inner world is split: the fantasy world of literature and writing which is reflected in his attitude to literature and literary play is hermetically sealed off from that of the rest of his inner world which is reflected in the despairing content of that literature. The fantasies of the first part can have nothing to do with the world of men: he admits to being a Platonist by condition, proceeding from the ideal to the object.[52] What becomes interesting is the constant assertion of the fantasy world of literature in the face of such an otherwise oppressive inner reality of schizoid despair. Sartre sees Genet in a similar situation—the fantasy world which he expresses through the process of writing *Our Lady of the Flowers* magically

50. Sartre, *Words*, p. 28.
51. Ibid., pp. 39-40.
52. Sartre, *Words*, p. 34.

transforms the thief into a poet. Or rather, there is another part of Genet which has lain dormant—the creative dynamic. Perhaps Sisyphus writes novels as he decends once again from the top of the hill.

Thus side by side with the messianic zeal of literature as salvation is the dread realization that literature will not and cannot transform the world; the world of political realities and the world of aesthetics are radically divorced. Yet the unshakable reality of the inner fantasy world generated in his grandfather's library can stand aloof, aside from the outer world—cynical and ironic—and art seems to be the only worthwhile reality.

Winnicott writes that play constitutes a third interconnecting area between the person and his environment.[53] Authentic play of course is good, and enjoyable in and for itself. But the play described by Sartre is not of this kind—it is empty and meaningless. Indeed, Sartre has an ironic vision of reality,[54] and this is the world *depicted* in his writing. I shall attempt to describe this ironic content further.

The ironic vision is a post-tragic one; the tragedy no longer matters. The tragic vision had constituted "an affirmation however negative of greatness in man".[55] There is no hope of redemption[56] and consciousness is a disease. Tragic visions lend meaning to a meaningless inevitable doom. Tragedy reveals its entanglement with the "unchartered background of man's humanity" which is beyond his control. But defiant if fruitless battle against the gods was an act of transcendence.[57] Tragedy involved character revelation and never development except toward a predestined fate.[58] A sense of doom arises at the very heart of success.[59] This sense of doom has developed to a situation in which no hope of the realization of values is possible for many writers who fall back on irony as "a necessary device to make the pain of life bearable". Irony is "an expression of metaphysical rebellion that knows its own futility".[60]

The lack of control we have of the consequences of our actions constitutes an irreducible figure. In an entirely alienated world in

53. D.W. Winnicott, *Playing and Reality*.
54. R. Schafer, "The Psychoanalytic Vision of Reality", *International Journal of Psychoanalysis*, 51 pp. 293-94. C. Glicksberg, *The Ironic Vision in Modern Literature*.
55. Glicksberg, *The Tragic Vision in Twentieth Century Literature*, p.5.
56. Ibid., p. 6.
57. L. Michel and R.B. Sewall (eds.), *Tragedy: Modern Essays in Criticism*, pp. 5, 6, 14-15.
58. Schopenauer cited in ibid., p. 38.
59. Ibid., p. 61.
60. Glicksberg, *The Tragic Vision*, p. 152.

which the individual is at the opposite polarity to community, the consequences of action of an individual are necessarily taken from him—hc has no control over them—yet this is so to some degree in any possible world. Oedipus freely pursues his life—and acts definitively for "right", "just" motives—yet he irrevocably does the opposite of what he intends—his mother cannot be restored for him. His "free" acts lead irresistibly to catastrophe.[61] This reflects something of the generality of the universe itself—we cannot control what we do. Causality and value are irredeemably estranged, with disastrous consequences for the agents. It is not accident—for this would merely be sad.[62]

Sartre has developed this horror so far that it is necessary to nullify it. We are radically divorced from the world—the in-itself and the for-itself have no meeting point. People often try and achieve an essence but deceive themselves, as the human condition is that of irreducible anxiety, a constant oscillation between varying forms of in-itself which we can never achieve—a frustrating but constant battle. If the battle cannot be won, why not give up the battle itself, pronounce the battle itself futile? Tired of frustration, we can withdraw from it altogether.

The century is one in which hopelessness is pervassive—post-tragic because it is beyond hope. Apathy is the stage beyond craving—when we know that wishing will not avail us any more.

*Altona* is, among other things, a play about this—men lock themselves up and cannot escape, tie themselves in knots from which they cannot extricate themselves. What is the point of acting when loser wins? We live, according to Sartre, in a world where violence is an irreducible and overwhelming force, in which individual transcendence is impossible since the individual is so conditioned by the group, by the world in which he has been brought up.

For Sartre, man is not what he is and is what he is not—he is the being whose being is always in question. Desiring to be God (who does not exist) he is conscious of his powerlessness. Actions militate against intention, and our own history seems out of our control. Authenticity and humanism are part of the *esprit de sérieux*. In politics, revolutionary organizations betray their mission—if the Communist Party is right, Sartre is more lonely than a madman, if it is wrong we are done for. The meaning of our lives may be determined by an instant—as in extreme situations such as torture. Everywhere we turn there is no exit, yet we seek some way out. In a

61. Michel and Sewall, *Tragedy*, p. 61.
62. *See* Jaspers in ibid.

godless universe, nothing ultimately matters. Neither Hitler's extermination camps, nor the cooling of the sun in 50,000 years time which will mean the extermination of the human race if it is still extant,[63] has any impact on an indifferent universe. Goetz tries to make God uneasy by deliberately doing wrong; then when he finds that evil is easy and good is impossible, he seeks to do good so as to be recognized by God. But he finds that God does not exist, and finally he resorts to the paradoxical world of action because there is no alternative left—his only way of being a nobody is to lead, his only way of loving is by hating, his only way of being benevolent is by destroying.[64] Sartrean man is without illusions about his place in the cosmos. He knows he is free—and even were God to exist this would make no difference to man's situation[65] since he could not be God.

Tragedy involved strong, powerful and overwhelmingly impassioned man confronting a relatively inevitable situation of despair. Whole, real, alive men faced situations beyond their control. Foretold and foredoomed, we see Oedipus unknowingly commit acts which spell out his fate. Characters majestically bestride the stage and their actions are part of a meaning which escapes them, yet exists and matters. People are joyous, happy, angry, sad, depressed, but not apathetic; what happens is of the greatest importance. Their existence itself is not at stake and life is anything but futile and hopeless. Life is eventful: the events belong to the actors who face the consequences with courage, cowardice, honour or treachery, but never with indifference or laughter at the nature of existence itself. Oedipus blinded himself; Pablo Iberta laughed so hard he cried.[66] Sartre is beyond tragedy; in the end it does not matter.

In the coldness of the death he faced, Pablo realized that his executioners "dolled up in their riding crops and boots were still going to die".[67] At the offer of a reprieve, Pablo still would not give away the true whereabouts of the man his executioners were searching, for now his life had no more value because "nothing was important".[68] Whether it was Pablo or Gris, now or later was of no consequence; now he understood the metaphysical absurdity of everything. He found the situation "somehow comic. It was obstinacy I thought, 'I

63. Sartre, *Words*, p. 155.f
64. Sartre, *The Devil and the Good Lord*, p. 149.f
65. Sartre, *Existentialism and Humanism*, p. 56, *The Flies*, p. 309, *Playboy* Interview, p. 169.f
66. Sartre (1937), "The Wall" in *Intimacy*, p. 73.
67. Ibid., p. 70.
68. Ibid.

must be stubborn'. And a droll sense of gaiety spread over me".[69]

Knowing that Gris was hiding at his cousin's, he decided to play a trick on the *falangistas*, and told them that Gris was hidden in the cemetery. He could scarcely control his laughter at the thought of the spectacle these grim and serious men would make lifting tombstones and opening vaults; it was "irresistibly funny".[70] On their return, Pablo is told they are not going to execute him. When he discovers that Gris had in fact been hiding in the cemetery, such was the irony of the situation that Pablo "laughed until I cried".[71] There is no tragedy here ... it simply does not matter. "The Wall" has put an end to tragedy, and with the death of tragedy goes the death of man. Having faced the wall nothing matters—all that remains is a cynical ironic enjoyment of the disrobing of serious man. The awareness of ironic twists provides tantalizing delight to the ironic soul. The ironic sould enjoys *play* and *plays* with words, situations—he can even play at being serious, but does not partake of the *esprit de sérieux* since he does not deceive himself that he is not playing.The game is the thing—individual actions do not count.

If the game is itself of no consequence, all that can matter is the play within it—an artistry for its own sake.[72] There seems to be some intrinsic pleasure in debunking, unveiling, showing the unimportance of something or somebody which was formerly assumed to be all-embracing in its significance. Perhaps the tables are turned; the ironic soul standing beyond the horizon outside history suddenly becomes a central focus in the significance of insignificance. The distance and unreality of the world to the man of irony is transmuted—the world itself is not seen in any greater depth of reality; what becomes real is its place in relation to the observer. The world is no longer outside, other: the cynic derives the only satisfaction allowed him by relating with it albeit in a narcissistic way. Mathieu decides to die to demonstrate the meaninglessness of living.[73] As Gorz writes, "if nothing has any importance, then the consciousness that nothing has any importance is of no importance".[74] Naturally that statement itself has no importance, and so on to infinity. Yet it is of the nature of irony that importance does not count as a "value"—everything becomes play: the only real measure to equal an indifferent and absurd reality is to be indifferent and absurd oneself. To take the absurd seriously is to submit, to fight the futile battle which one can

69. Ibid., p. 70.
70. Ibid., p. 72.
71. Ibid., p. 73.
72. L. Trilling, *Sincerity and Authenticity*, p. 100.
73. *See* Ch. 2.
74. A. Gorz, *The Traitor*, p. 180.

never win. Not to participate at all, to stand aloof, distant and untouched—this is to win. In *Morts sans sépulture*, the aim is to win so that one will have that at least. Sartre might call this the sin of "pride",[75] but what else can a man do in the situation—except laugh as in "The Wall" (on which *Morts sans sépulture* is modelled). Either way something exists—something eyes the world with some being which is not the world. Dismissal and total negation are the barest—the deepest in the sense that there is no place further down. The sense of absolute isolation and futility is precisely a state of no care—former cares seem so ridiculous. Tragedy is now absurd; nothing can touch the ironic soul so there is nothing left to fear. The satisfaction lies in an activity which leaves him something to laugh *at* to define his existence. The ironic soul without paradox is like a fish without water. His laughter is the final defence against annihilation. This is perhaps a reason that it is so important for Sartre to demythologize, to reveal "bad faith" for something replaces "bad faith"—irony, absurdity, our original state of anxiety. The ironic soul is not engulfed and in his total powerlessness against absurdity, there lies—paradoxically—an infinite omnipotence. He has faced the Absurd, and laughed in its face—he has seen through it, and rejected or discarded it—everything. With schizoid suicide, the worst signs are not where the person feels most depressed and hurt—the real danger is when this state is passed beyond into the realm of indifference to everything. This is frequently where the ironic emerges most clearly—and most dangerously. The schizoid drifts into death as if it were merely another trivial action.

"Life begins on the other side of despair", avers Orestes. Before man gods are powerless since this is his freedom[76]—the ironic soul finds he is nothing—that there is a final sense of triviality in doom. Orestes relieves Argos of its flies (scarcely grand objects) by taking their weight upon himself. If the flies represent the sins of the Argyles, the Argyles are a hapless people, cowered into self-abasement and capable of no nobility. By ridding them of the curse of the flies, Orestes does not make a truly grand gesture—as the Argyles seem not to "deserve" it.

In any case, Orestes takes the burden upon himself for himself and not for the Argyles. It is to bring him to the ground, and to find a sense of belonging. Ironically this can be done only in exile—his motives are purely personal. His defiance of the gods brings a final triviality; he is empty, nothing, a great void. There is no substan-

75. Contat and Rybalka, p. 134.
76. Sartre, *The Flies*, p. 309.

tiality to his soul. Freedom came down like a thunderbolt, and he knew what he was—nothing. The freedom that man gains is his loss: he is free for nothing. We are never given a glimpse by Sartre of how life might begin on the other side of despair—what it would be like.

Why is there not such a glimpse of a free life in Sartre's work? We do not find any forays of authentic love in Sartre's work—the closest are perhaps in some of the incestuous relationships he describes. Hilda shows little sign of loving Goetz—she needs to do good and be recognized. Brunet and Vicarios achieve some form of closeness only in the unfinished fourth volume of *The Roads to Freedom*. Women play no enviable part in Sartre's works, nor does sex appear to be anything but odious. The men depicted seem to be mere shadows and the general mood provides no possibility of authentic relationship.[77]

The quest for the absolute and immortality through literature has been an important theme for Sartre—it replaces religion in a godless world. Literature had been seen by Sartre as a magically powerful sword to slash through the mystifications of a terrible world, but more latterly he has seen it as impotent in terms of its ability to transform the world. He had seen literature as providing a world through which he could exist, as communists and Christians could see themselves as soldiers of the Party and the Church respectively. The choice to become a writer involved the choice of more than a simple vocation: it was the choice of a life-project. There has always been a tension between the worlds of the imaginary and of action for Sartre, and they can be seen to be radically split, especially lately into literature and direct political action. Words throughout Sartre's life have had a magical quality about them and seem to occupy an autonomous existence. This is perhaps an instance of the impact of advanced techological societies on a language that seems wrenched from the realities it putatively describes. And the realities themselves present an ambiguous aspect since the consequences of action seem so paradoxically related with the actions themselves. Sartre the intellectual, the writer, the bastard who stands on the edges of the worlds of the bourgeoisie and the working class without properly belonging to either, can see all this very clearly. Writing seems politically useless in the first world where its critical content is mediated and transformed into merchandise; in the second in which this content scarcely appears and in which there has been such degeneration that revolution from within is out of the question; and in the third world where metaphysics takes a poor second place to the political struggle to secure a minimally human material existence.

77. S. Lilar, *A propos de Sartre et de l'amour*, Ch. 4. K. Stern, *The Flight from Woman*, Ch. 7.

As I have argued, words which appear so inherently powerful in phantasy seem to be alarmingly impotent in reality. The intellectual whose profession is words often has problems of feeling his own reality, of distinguishing dream from actuality, of constant doubt and uncertainty about everything which seems somehow to elude him. For Sartre action appears to involve submergence in an organization and a relatively unconditional acceptance of an ideology: this is the opposite of the writer's duty. Sartre's solution to the problems of words and action was through the notion of commitment in literature, and this he pursued with the messianic zeal of a religion. But he was not successful, and the content of his thought was opposed to the possibility of a valuable commitment. Further, literature was later seen by Sartre as only one step in the process of communication and he could see that the writer could not control what happened to his work once it was published. It is possible to understand his fear of institutionalization in this light. Literature in a society which co-opts it perhaps becomes an impotent Sisyphean defiance. When Sartre became "converted" to a membership of society, literature lost much of this defiance and Sartre became absorbed in his largest work ever, located in the world of the imaginary, while at the same time becoming involved in a spontaneous politics of Sisyphean defiance.

Sartre's engrossment in literature may then be understood in a psychoanalytic way: Sartre could pour out the pure milk of paradise instead of being reliant on the tasteless and nauseating milk that he finds in the outer world. Literature, for Sartre, is a form of play and while reality is seen ironically, everybody plays at being what he is not in our world of radical alienation. But Sartre has a part of himself which is firmly detached from it, living in the world generated by that of his grandfather's library and his original choice to become a writer. This private inner world of artistic fantasy has sufficient autonomy to allow Sartre to see the post-tragic world in which man seems to be dead.

Thus the world which Sartre describes in his literature is that of a prison from which there is no escape. All we can do is involve ourselves in meaningless and ironic play which is far from the image of fulfilling and intrinsically enjoyable play. If prison and play are indeed the major themes of writers who describe the world from outside it, Sartre is an excellent example of this. One part of his inner world remains locked away in the recesses of the image of his grandfather's library and enjoys a form of play in his inner world, while for the rest, Sartre's vision is an ironic one of the human condition—an unbarred cage in which play is only shadow-boxing.

# 4

# Recognition and Politics

For Sartre our existence is irremediably bound up with that of others. It is not a question of social contract that the individual makes with others in renouncing certain individual pleasures so as to derive the benefits of community. Solipsism is never a question since I find the other before I find myself - indeed I find myself through the other. Thus the mode of my existence is dependent on the other. Hegel's Master-Slave dialectic is taken up and "existentialized" by Sartre (through Kojève) in such a way that the struggle for recognition by the other is of paramount importance in our concrete relations with others. The original state of being does not lie for Sartre in an "I-Thou" dialogic relationship; it resides rather in that of original conflict. What I need most - the security of being regarded as a subject by another subject - is unfortunately exactly what cannot be guaranteed since the subjectivity of the other involves constant choice, and therefore implies the ever-present possibility of rejection. For if this possibility is not allowed, then the look of the other is not that of a free subject. A pledge once made involves loss of subjectivity since one is being loved not for oneself now, but because of the pledge. Since I am a *nothingness* I have no security in my own foundations and seek it through others who, similarly placed, seek theirs through me. Our inextricable dependence on others for our own self-image is primary. The joy in love, when there is joy, Sartre assures us, is simply that we feel our existence to be justified after all.

While the Hegelian Master-Slave dialectic is finally transcended in the absolute unity which is that of the World-Spirit as Being-in-and-for-itself, Sartrean man has no such luck. Alienation in the irreducible duality which is our existence is the unhappy consciousness of the Cartesian philosopher in a world without God. I am at the mercy of the other who constitutes my existence. If he lets me control him. then any security his look seems to offer me is false since it consists of my own reflection of what I want to be rather than what I am. When I enter a collusive relationship with another, there is the constant possibility of a third looking on and seeing through the sham. It is my awareness of the possibility of the awareness that makes collusion finally fruitless in gaining security. The inner feeling —or at least fear—of being *de trop* is always present.[1]

If this situation is not sufficiently disheartening, the discovery of forces which operate unknown and beyond, yet through my relations with the other provides for still greater disappointment. For the second world war was only the final resultant of obscure and collective forces which had, in fact, been governing people's lives for a long time without their knowing it. Even the most private actions could be seen as historically mediated.[2] The condition of an apolitical and "free" life which was unconnected with the past—or even present realities—was itself a result of bourgeois conditioning.[3] History situates and flows in on us whether we like it or not.[4] The war had effected a decisive conversion for Sartre since through it he realized that we are always politically situated and from his camp experience learned that solidarity with others counted as a possibility.[5] Not only were present and past political forces important, but Sartre began to discover the importance of the past of the individual. Our area of choice began to diminish quite drastically as the forces of the collective and individual past entered the horizon; the disowning of these realities was itself a product of them. As the truth seemed increasingly to constitute the whole, the individual seemed increasingly constituted by a vast conglomerate of intermeshed groups. Sartre began to see psychoanalysis and Marxism as essential tools for explaining our existence - without however abandoning his former categories. Indeed Marxism needed to be existentialized.[6]

*Critique de la raison dialectique* concentrated on group behaviour as fundamental. An individual could only be understood in terms of the groups to which he belonged knowingly and unknowingly. "Pledged" and "serial" groups were ineradicable determinants of individual existence. Scarcity was our universal condition, and thus there is bound to be conflict. While the category or "scarcity" may well have replaced that of "nothingness", the same primacy of the

1. Sartre, *Being and Nothingness*, Part Three.
2. Sartre, *What is Literature?*, p. 157.
3. de Beauvoir, *The Prime of Life*, p. 21.
4. Sartre, *What is Literature?*, pp.156-57.
5. de Beauvoir, *Force of Circumstance*, p. 13.
6. Sartre, *Search for a Method*, Ch. 1.

lack is present; while the *pour-soi* was replaced by praxis, the self seems to have lost still more power, and where the *pratico-inerte* is substituted for the *en-soi*, the same primitive division remains.

Whether or not the theory embodied in the *Critique* is Marxist, it is certainly a Sartrean one.[7] Hope of redemption seems further than ever before, for the possibility of intervention of a "third" force to save the world seems more remote than ever, given the dominance of truly alienated group praxes which seems to assume autonomous existences. More than ever the individual appears to depend on the groups to which he belongs to achieve an identity. For terror and violence are the frightening consequences of violating group norms - and there can be nowhere else to go for the ostracized individual whose identity is fused with that of his group. The first important mediating group the child encounters is that of the family, but this is only a certain way of living the culture at large. While not reducible to the latter the mode of being of the family is conditioned by the culture. Generalized attitudes towards oneself and others are culturally determined and "reality" is socially constructed, as are such concepts as "normal" and "good". Entwined in a vast network of interweaving groups, the individual finds great difficulty in finding himself through the others through whom Sartrean man must find his identity. Recognition becomes virtually impossible unless it is equated with conformity to the rules, norms, wishes and expectations of others. Certainly love is impossible, and unity is constituted in hating the same enemy.

This could be seen as relatively simple in the Republic of Silence of the war years, but the choices have become increasingly difficult - indeed Sartre states that he did not complete *The Roads to Freedom* because the political choices were far more difficult than during the war.[8] Extreme situations in which there is a simple choice can provide a situation in which a person might achieve the recognition of the other which he so desperately needs. For the pre-war Roquentin was outside it all—and there was no hope of entry into the human world. The only exit from his own was through art—and that in a book which would be as "hard as steel" and which would make people "ashamed of their existence".[9] Another Sartrean character, Paul Hilbert, finds recognition impossible, and his way of being recognized is to make people recognize him by the act of killing some of their number.[10] Lucien Fleurier who, like Roquentin and

7. Cranston, "Sartre and Violence", p. 23. R. Aron, *Marxism and the Existentialists*, p. 10.
8. "Sartre talks to Tynan", II. de Beauvoir, *Force of Circumstance*, p. 206.
9. Sartre, *Nausea*, p. 252.
10. Sartre, "Erostratus".

Hilbert, sees himself as nothing and the world as nauseous, finds recognition by assuming the identity of "a person who hates Jews".[11] Mathieu, who is a continuation of the character Roquentin[12], shares a similar problematic in *The Age of Reason*, and in *The Reprieve* goes "sheeplike" to the war. Neither Mathieu nor Lucien seems especially interested in the rights and wrongs of politics; they are primarily concerned with identity. Lucien happens upon the *Action Francaise* which conveniently offers him a reality: he is defined in terms of his negative relations with Jews. No question of the validity of these views ever arises for Lucien: he simply wants to **be** someone, just as Hilbert does. Had he been German, Mathieu could as easily have gone sheeplike in the Nazi army call-up as so many Germans did in their otherwise rootless condition. Mathieu, Lucien, Hilbert are children of the century as were the Germans of the period who did not wish to bear the burden of freedom in a Europe in which great changes and traumata had occurred since the beginning of this century.

The characters in *Altona* are all condemned. The Father collaborated with Hitler for his own ends—he sold the Nazis some land in which to build a concentration camp. But he regarded his cooperation as of no political significance; indeed there were at most three dozen criminals he says.[13] When the Father informed on a Polish Rabbi whom Franz was hiding and the SS beat the Rabbi to death in front of Franz, Franz went to the front with a vengeance and took on dangerous assignments partly to expiate his father's guilt by his own death. However he had succeeded in these missions and was decorated in front of the entire army—loser wins. Later when Germany was obviously losing the war, he turned his aggression to a group of prisoners, and soon became the butcher of Smolensk. "It is because you're an informer that I'm a torturer", Franz tells his father. But this was not wholly true - Franz had despised and felt contempt for the prisoners he had seen in the concentration camp built on the land his father had sold the Nazis; he had not felt sorry for them. In this as in all else he was the shadow of his father - he was destined to repeat his father's past, and to be head of the firm which ruled him. But Franz locked himself up after the war so as to take the guilt of the Germans on his shoulders and bear witness for the century. This is it—a world in which technology has been used so

11. Sartre, "The Childhood of a Leader" in *Intimacy*, p. 216. Sartre (1946), *Portrait of the Anti-Semite*.
12. Sartre quoted in Contat and Rybalka, p. 114.
13. Sartre, *Altona*, p. 35.

destructively, in which people are loathe to bear the burden of responsibility for their actions, and in which the nation that lost the war leads Europe. Where is the morality here?

*Altona* can be understood on a number of levels. On a personal level Franz achieved a moment of independence when he tortured the prisoners. He had freely taken on the identity of the aggressor, and he tortured for no reason except the horror he could strike. He was gratuitously torturing people to make them submit to him. In a life in which he had felt so helpless and impotent, a weak nonentity, he could become a terrifying somebody. Germany however had lost the war and won the peace. The German people were not punished though they seemed responsible. As Heinrich assures Goetz who does evil so as "to make the Almighty uneasy" thus recognizing him, it is very easy to do evil. In fact, everyone does evil and no one does good.[14] Even Franz's maniacal torturing was insignificant in the face of the rejuvenation of the German nation — even his only "independent" act was not too significant. Sartre writes of the obsessive presence of future centuries today, and Franz bears witness to our time by recognizing and even accepting the guilt of its enormous destructiveness. At least some sense of justice might prevail. But where loser wins, we are robbed of ourselves. For Franz there is no way of accepting himself as any self at all in a wealthy Germany: he is a pawn in a mad world.

Nothing makes sense when our actions inevitably have the opposite consequences from those intended—Franz is impotent. In the world upstairs, he could phantasize and rationalize the oppressive weight of the century's destructiveness before the tribunal of the future: men owned their actions and could be judged for them. But Franz discovers the opposite to be true and this denies him any reality of his own. Franz was nothing but the product of the marriage of his father and the firm. But the Father finally takes all the guilt and responsibility for everything, and with this Franz himself is to disappear into his father and they die as one. Franz's future was mapped out at birth as was the Father's—the firm, as a symbol of the results of all our actions had taken on a reality of its own, one which finally destroyed its creators. In this radically alienated world, the concept of recognition as anybody, the concept of any form of autonomy has no meaning. The actions of Franz can be understood as seeking such an identity—but so fruitlessly that suicide remains the only way out. Father has lost any authority he ever had and the child is doomed to be nothing, weak and impotent in a world of

14. Sartre, *The Devil and the Good Lord*, p. 63.

monstrous constructions which now control him.

*Altona* shares the landscape of the *Critique*, and there is little or no room to move. Our choices are made for us whether we seem to choose or not. Given the inverse congruence of what we will and what we do, no recognition or meeting is possible between people who are inevitably robbed of their actions. A feeling of self is impossible in a world in which the self as distinct from a collection of roles does not exist—apathy prevails. The groups to which the individual belongs have taken over entirely and constitute the individual. Treachery, injustice, criminality are the lot of the flesh-eating beasts of the modern world: yet these people proclaim the value of justice, equality, freedom and dignity. The scapegoat Genet achieves a liberation by deliberately assuming the role given him, and then transforming the criminal into a writer. Franz has no such alternative.

The story of Franz is biographical, constantly moving between private and public psychological and political realities. By no means is an exclusively "psychological" explanation in order, since the internalization of the external much prevails over the externalization of the internal. Franz could preserve a semblance of freedom shut up in his room, the phantasy system of his inner world, but when the outside world enters in the form of Johanna, it is shattered. And Johanna discovers in the world of Franz that "there's only one truth - the horror of living".[15] But there can be no retreat for Johanna into Franz's world. For Leni, who can act as representative of the outer and inner worlds, can act as a third party to destroy their relationship by representing the outer world; just as Johanna had done to that of Franz and Leni. When the Father says, "A family is a house",[16] he can be seen to be referring to the family constituting a phantasy system. If this is disturbed from outside, if it is seen for what it is, it crumbles. Yet if it crumbles, there is nothing left but annihilation, so Leni finally takes the only other way out—she shuts herself up in Franz's room and lies to herself, for it is the only way of living in an otherwise unlivable situation. The strong, according to the Father, do nothing and live in close intimacy with death.[17] Franz, Johanna, Leni and the Father are strong and see reality while Werner is weak and conforms. The strong, for Sartre, are prepared to look for the truth. But in *Altona* facing reality is distinctly non-adaptive—it is a sign of the madness of the modern world.

After the collapse of Nazi Germany the identification of the

15. Sartre, *Altona*, p. 111.
16. Idem.
17. Ibid., p. 31.

masses with the Nazis ceased and the memory virtually extinguished. The regime had failed to continue to provide the milk and honey to the masses whose ties were pre-Oedipal. These other directed people could not defend basic trust against basic mistrust. Mitscherlich points out:

> Having never experienced firm object ties, the other-directed individual is an opportunist not out of weakness of character, but because his character development has never attained stability. He is governed by pre-Oedipal wishes, external stimuli without being able to organize these into a memory, in the sense of a consciousness, a self. He lives by the feeling of the moment in accordance with the all-or-nothing law of stimulus and reaction, just as a suckling lives between hunger and satiety.

The other-directed individual is not capable of immediate renunciation for an ultimate goal. In Germany,

> he still sees the world in terms of a power-impotence relationship, the only one he has truly experienced, and has never reached the stage of discovering the possibility of independent thought. Therefore, instead of exercising the latter, he projects outside himself responsibility for behaviour which suddenly turns out to have been guilty. It is the Fuhrer who should be held responsible, he says, not the obedient children of the state who merely carried out his orders.

It can be added that whereas the inner-directed man needed democracy as a framework for the "expression of his values, interests and ideas, the other-directed man does not need it". Mitscherlich cites Dahrendorf:

> He needs society and as long as society gives him the guidance and security he cannot find in himself, the political institutions under which he lives are a matter of relative indifference to him.[18]

This well illustrates the world of *Altona*. The first problem is the search for an identity in the all-or-nothing world of power and impotence. Franz is defending himself against an overwhelming feeling of impotence in a world in which basic trust is not possible. Things have overridden persons, and their fate seems to have little to do with their intentions. It is only in Oedipal and post-Oedipal situations that a sufficient sense of secure selfhood which is adequate to take on the problems of the external world with any realism and power can exist. But where secure object-relations have not existed in the family or in society at large, the quest for security overrides every other question—including the rightness or wrongness of political issues —

18. A. Mitscherlich, *Society Without the Father: A Contribution to Social Psychology*, pp. 284-6.

since the life of the person is at stake. Thus we can see that in an analysis of *Altona* the "political" problem of Nazism is a symptom of the kind of culture which not only preceded it but existed during and after it. But it can also be seen that the overwhelming power of the machine seems to have crushed the possibilities of collective autonomy. The "weak", like Werner, conform to prescribed roles and fit in with the prevailing order without ever questioning it. The "strong", like Franz, try to achieve some form of independence where this is impossible, and are finally absorbed and come to nothing. It can be seen that the basic thread of the play is not so much concerned with the rights and wrongs of political realities as with our ability to attain an identity in the face of an engulfing world which is mediated through politics, business, family, ideology and so on.

The basic problems of Franz, Goetz, Mathieu, Lucien, Hugo, and Roquentin are those which reflect on and through the political and psychological planes, yet which concern the ability of modern man to preserve any self at all. The recognition they all seek is impossible since the relationships depicted never presuppose the integrity of the people concerned, and indeed point to the constant problems of achieving an identity within relations in which basic trust between persons in their own right simply does not exist. Politics and the cause are secondary. If Mathieu could have been Franz, so could Brunet have been a soldier of the Third Reich instead of the P.C.F. Franz shuts himself up against this world.

The basic cultural situations of these characters were similar in a century in which Western man struggles to keep going in the face of enormous change, and the awareness and impotence that influence it in a world in which he feels abandoned. The external has been introjected to such an extent that no prospect of autonomy is even a viable alternative. The externalizations and internalizations are so confused in the other-directed man fixated at pre-Oedipal stages of development that politics and psychology become fused, with the analysis of the individual being seen more and more in terms of functions of immensely powerful social modalities. If Sartre's characters seem to be stick figures struggling with the problem of having any identity of their own at all, and if the relationships they are engaged in are mainly of the oral or narcissistic types, it is because they never have had the possibility open to them of authentic relating.

The closest relationships are exhibited in torture. The fascination which Sartre has with torture (discussed in Ch. 1) is partly related to the possibility in it of recognition. Franz's only independent actions were in torturing people. Where there is no feeling of personal autonomy, the only feeling of having a self can come in a fight to the death with someone else. According to Sartre (as with Camus) we are all either victims or executioners and we can only escape being one by taking on the role of the other.[19] Pure evil shines forth "in the close and almost sexual relation between the executioner and his victim. For torture is first of all a matter of debasement". It is the victim in this battle who decides when and if to give in.[20] The man who talks "becomes one with his executioner. Coupled as man and wife, these two lovers made the abject night terrible".[21] The victim may be a "groaning, sweating, filthy creature who begs for mercy and abandons himself in a swooning consent with the moanings of an amorous woman who yields everything", but the executioner knows that he is bearing down on himself as well for the victim is an aspect of himself. When the victim speaks he tells all, since the only way of enduring his hatred is to hate all mankind including himself. The executioner and victim are of one accord since the torturer has "symbolically gratified his hatred of mankind".[22]

The indissoluble partnership of torturer and victim is for Sartre the ultimate form of recognition. Indeed the torturer pits himself against the tortured for his "manhood" and the dual is fought as if it were not possible for both sides to belong to the human race.[23] As has been seen in Ch. 1, the victim winning means the end of the torturer's lordship. Henri Alleg had not seen torture as a means of drawing a confession (*un aveu*) out of him.[24] The French term also means the recognition by a vassal of lordship. Thus torture is seen by Sartre as a struggle for recognition, as the master-slave dialectic in action. We can resist suffering to death and beat the torturers by not submitting to them. A victory is possible for the man who, by refusing to give in, turns the tables on his torturers. This struggle is most real and the hatred the torturer and his victim manifest for each other is absolute recognition. For example, Lucie feels closer to her torturer than to her lover. She wants them to come again and torture her so that she can refuse to submit once again.[25] When the victim wins, he becomes a witness to the ignominy of his torturers.[26] He is witnessed by them as victor, as absolute in his power to undergo anything, in an affirmation that it is possible to be recognized as human in the most

19. Sartre, "A Victory", p. 13.
20. Sartre, *What is Literature?*, pp. 160-61.
21. Sartre, "A Victory", p. 13.
22. Sartre, *What is Literature?*, p. 161.
23. Sartre, "A Victory", p. 23.
24. Sartre, "La Réponse d'Henri Alleg".
25. Sartre, *Men Without Shadows*, p. 214.
26. Sartre, "La Réponse d'Henri Alleg".

horrific and nightmarish circumstances. The irreducible evil of the torturers is conquered by the man who resists them. The freedom under the Occupation was solidarity in hating the same enemy.[27] But also there was a total responsibility vested in the man in the total solitude of the torture chamber.[28]

It is this image of ourselves as both torturer and victim that Sartre wants to convey: "Torturer and victim, always it is we, the police who are giving the traitor the third degree".[29] The only mode of transcendence is by not giving in to the torturers, internal or external, thus substituting a new set of values for the old so that it becomes clear that man is free.[30] Sartre sees torture as a "plague infecting our whole era" in which "Hitler was only a forerunner".[31] It infects all of us whether we like it or not and "the blinding sun of torture is at its zenith; it lights up the whole country".[32]

Sartre had argued in *Saint Genet* that the criminal and the saint constituted an "eternal couple". Sartre sees evil in others as a mirror we may hold up to ourselves - all relationships are sado-masochistic. Each of us incarnates our culture and what happens even in the colonies are externalizations of ourselves that we do not normally accept:

> Our victims know us by their scars and by their chains, and it is this that makes their evidence irrefutable. It is enough that they show us what we have made of them for us to realize what we have made of ourselves.[33]

The third world becomes a terrifying screen on which we can see ourselves if we look. We can see the "normal" person become a malicious torturer, the unwilling conscript become a relentless murderer. Sartre is pointing to what we should know from the experiences of Nazi Germany: respectable and normal people can and do perform the most vicious atrocities. This can happen because we can project our own aggression, hatred and disapprobation on to appropriate objects. With little coercion, the "normal", law-abiding, other-directed person of our civilization will perform the most barbarous acts. The barbarism of civilization is no accident; it is an intrinsic part of it, as Freud saw with alarming clarity:[34] for Sartre

27. Sartre, "Merleau-Ponty", p. 231. Sartre, *The Devil and the Good Lord*, p. 145.
28. Sartre, "Paris Alive: The Republic of Silence".
29. Sartre, "Of Rats and Men", p. 344.
30. Ibid., p. 15.
31. Ibid., p. 20.
32. Sartre (1961), Preface to F. Fanon, *The Wretched of the Earth*, p. 25.
33. Ibid., p. 12.
34. S. Freud, "Reflections Upon War and Death" and "Why War" in P. Rieff (ed.) *Sigmund Freud: Character and Culture*.

extreme situations of torture are our ordinary situations taken to their limit. The "third" world may now react against the torturers of the first, and to a lesser extent the second world.

> If the European eventually brings himself to hate his own face, it will be because it is reflected by an Arab. In looking at these two indissoluble partnerships, the colonizer and the colonized, the executioner and his victim, we can see that the second is only an aspect of the first.

The executioners are not the colonizers nor vice verse. Most of the executioners have never thought about the war. "But hate is a magnetic field: it has crossed over to them, corroded them and enslaved them".[35]

The hatred that the victims of the third world bear for those of the Western world can be understood within the relationship of torture. Sartre can see that meaning can be real for the people of the third world in common struggle against the evil inroads of the West. The third world may yet preserve humanity as Europe has destroyed it, the wretched of the earth may yet overthrow their colonizers and institute a new world. Sartre's enthusiasm for China and Cuba exhibit this concern. But what happens if and when they win? Against whom will they fight then? Will they not then degenerate as the U.S.S.R. did some time after the 1917 revolution? Will not the same problem of group terror exist? While there is a force which they may fight, it is possible for the third world to recognize itself. While there is not enough food or shoes, metaphysical problems need not trouble the rising nations. Revolutionary intellectuals would not write metaphysics, nor in all probability read Robbe-Grillet or Sartre.[36] But their very ascendancy would spell out their doom. Sado-masochistic relations and widespread feelings of futility will prevail in their turn; the world of torture is that of recognition.

The world itself seems to be a torture house, a vast prison, a concentration camp. It seems to be the "closed system run on hate" that Fairbairn and Guntrip describe.[37] The closeness of the embraces of torturer and victim which Sartre describes can be seen as it was in Sartre's Hell; as a defence against the feeling of being nothing at all; the feeling of going nowhere, of being dead. As long as there is someone somewhere to fight against and to be recognized by, a future seems possible. But in point of fact, this future is plainly illusion since it exists within the framework of sado-masochistic relationships. There seems no authentic transcendence - one which

35. Sartre, "A Victory", p. 26.
36. Sartre, "A Long Bitter-Sweet Madness". In fact Sartre has recently become disillusioned with Cuba.
37. *See* Ch. 2.

would be positive and revolutionary instead of rebellious; for the rebel needs the object he attacks to achieve an identity. The revolutionary may, however, transcend the old structures towards a future whose promise lies in self-realization. But for Sartre, this is impossible: there is never a self to realize. On the contrary, man is negativity, lack—the world into which he is thrown and abandoned deprives him of fulfilment. Scarcity prevails and conflict is the necessary mode of being-for-others. The Western world which so controls its inhabitants may in fact contain or buy off the third—the world of tyrants and tyranized, of colonists and colonized constitutes both the inner and outer worlds. But decolonization may well bring with it for the colonized an ultimate sense of futility, for sense and meaning could only be attained in a struggle to the death based on hatred.

Conflict has always characterized existentialist political life as an aspect of the structure of being-for-others. There was never any danger of Sartre being a reformist—a literature of extreme situations could scarcely allow that.[38] For Sartre, since our hell is other people who torture each other, the likelihood of an amicable resolution is nil.

Sartre's epic, *The Devil and the Good Lord*, mirrors Sartre's own political evolution.[39] All is conflict whether the duel is with the Lord or with the oppressive forces of mankind. In either case Goetz's struggle is for recognition by any means. the cause for which he fights is immaterial. He would destroy the city of Worms and massacre its inhabitants to make God uneasy, deafen Him and crucify Him as his only worthy enemy. Mankind was irrelevant;[40] when he finds that it is not evil but good that is impossible to do, he creates a City of the Sun, so as to be a saint instead of a criminal. But his saintliness is not for the sake of the achievement of good, but simply so that he himself would be recognized by God. "What will become of me if you take away my means of doing good?" he desperately asks.[41] But he had in fact worsened the lot of the peasants he supposed himself to be helping.[42] Of course, this was because the peasants were for Goetz only an instrument with which to help himself by showing God that he could do the impossible, that he could do Good purely.

All along humanity was cast aside to reach God. Only God existed - man was an optical illusion. According to Goetz, man was made to

38. Burnier, *Choice of Action*, pp. 24-25.
39. de Beauvoir, *Force of Circumstance*, p. 254.
40. Sartre, *The Devil and the Good Lord*, p. 83.
41. Ibid., p. 71.
42. Heinrich to Goetz: "In one day of virtue you killed more people than in thirty-five years of malice", ibid., p. 138. *See also* ibid., pp. 72-75, 112 ff, 139.

destroy the man in himself. Goetz would henceforth chastize man's sins in his own disgusting flesh. To conquer himself he deliberately gave himself temptations so as to refuse and overcome them. As with the saints of old, the only way of loving him was then to torture him, to deprive him. This was of course so that he could feel real: one half of him was the accomplice against the other half. This is an inner sado-masochistic torture house of his own creation, again a system run on hate. How different is this from the previous system when he did evil? In that period, the bastard Goetz was a traitor by choice who hated himself, who perpetrated the greatest evils imaginable so as to catch the eye of God. God hates him, therefore, Goetz exists. However, he can never quite convince himself of God's hatred, and perpetrates progressively greater atrocities so as to achieve recognition. But there are never any thunderbolts for God does not even notice him. Even in a wager with God, Goetz cheats in the throw of the dice. The ultimate fear the bastard has is that of being ignored by indifferent others, for he does not recognize himself, and has an inordinate need of the notice of others. He will be good or evil, so long as he is recognized as something.

For Goetz, to exist is to exist in the eyes of God, and human beings are simply the raw material with which Goetz fashions his encounter with God. He does not seek relation with them—he is alone and they are his instruments. This is so as much in Goetz the criminal as in Goetz the saint—they both want to be recognized by the significant other and the means are purely subsidiary. The alternatives are not good and evil, but being recognized as something or being nothing. This problematic is made abundantly clear in *Saint Genet* which chronicles the evolution of Genet which so resembles that of Goetz and of Sartre himself.

When Goetz realizes that his efforts for evil and good have been in vain, since everyone else does evil too and his efforts to do good have turned out to have the opposite effect, Goetz wonders why God will not permit him to become and do good, while implanting in Goetz such a strong desire to do so.[43] Good was only possible after he was evil and when he tried to achieve good it disappeared elusively like a mirage. Why?[44]

The answer is not difficult, for at no stage did Goetz *give* anything. As Goetz himself realizes, he gave nothing away but merely read a public declaration when he handed his lands over to the peasants. Possessions shrivel in his hands. He had never possessed anything

43. Ibid., p. 140.
44. Idem.

since possession is a "friendliness between man and objects".[45] There is an immense difference between a mechanical act for some ulterior motive and a genuine gift. Laing notes the difference between being *passed* a cup of tea in a "tea ceremonial" and being *given* one as one person to another person.[46] As with the schizoid who feels the same abandonment, the bastard feels bereft of relationship and life becomes a desperate series of ploys, manoeuvres and play acting to manufacture a semblance of being any kind of person at all.[47] Bastards are nothing and have nothing. Goetz sees the world through the keyhole as an outsider. It is a "neat little egg neatly packed where everything fits into the place God assigned it".[48] He does not want to be loved, since it gives the lover all the pleasure; he is an unalloyed monster or saint with evil or good his reason for living.[49] He has always been divided in two, each half horrified with the other half. In his struggle for recognition Goetz never did evil to hurt people or good to help them. These actions were performed not as ends in themselves where people are treated as ends in themselves, but for Goetz's own narcissistic gratification. Thus Goetz characterizes himself as an idealist in that he strives for ideals rather than real change. But the ideals are not for mankind—or even the poor whom he so detests.[50] Indeed his "good" is destructive, and he concludes that he gave only to destroy. Before he had violated souls with torture, now he did so with "good".[51] It could not really be otherwise since the surest way of not achieving good (as with pleasure) is to pursue it. Good and pleasure lie in the fulfilment of goals: they are not the goals themselves. When men are not loved for themselves but for what we would like them to be or give us, this is a certain way of harming them and ourselves. No real relationship is involved, and idealism is often a facade for narcissistic idealization.[52] This is clearly the case with Goetz - his fencing with God manifests the projection of his own inner conflicts on to the world as a battlefield.

But Goetz finally realizes that God does not exist since it was impossible to do good without having the opposite effect. God is the absence, the loneliness of man. Goetz "killed" God because He divided him from mankind. But His death isolated Goetz still more.

45. Sartre, *The Devil and the Good Lord*, p. 137.
46. Laing (1969), *Self and Others*, p. 106.
47. Guntrip, *Psychoanalytic Theory*, p. 149.
48. Sartre, *The Devil and the Good Lord*, p. 33.
49. Ibid., pp. 46, 55.
50. Ibid., p. 138.
51. Ibid.
52. S. Freud, "On Narcissism" in *General Psychological Theory*.

If God was dead why is Goetz so alone?[53] Is it because he had never entered relationships with others, had he never had any but narcissistic gratifications? He feels different from the rest of men, and feels he would poison them by relating with them;[54] his love he feels is destructive, a typical schizoid fear. If God as significant other does not exist, if he cannot be self-sufficient, and if it is impossible to relate with men without destroying them or himself, then Goetz feels he does not exist; he is nothing.[55] In desperation he takes the step of asking Nasti the peasant leader if he can join the peasant army as a private. "Nasti, allow me to be a nobody."[56] He will be a man among men but undifferentiated from them; submerged and engulfed. Nasti will not accept this and forces Goetz to lead the army. But Goetz will not acknowledge that he is leading it—he receives his orders from elsewhere![57] Goetz will not be able to relate with anyone and the kingdom of man begins for Geotz with a murder: he will be a hangman and a butcher.[58] Victory will be assured only when his men fear him more than they do the enemy. He will make men hate him since he has no other way of loving them; he will be cruel to be kind, he will destroy to love, and will be alone under an empty sky since God does not exist.[59] This is resignation rather than hope, for love as well as hate is seen as destructive.

Goetz will suffer all his life from the death of God, the death of sense and meaning. There is certainly no indication that he will accept human relationships with any form of spontaneity. He can only live for the sake of some form of idealization or because he is obliged to act in a certain way. He cannot accept Hilda's love (itself like Goetz's not based on reciprocity) and he can only relate by destroying. Since he does not love himself, how can he love others? Goetz is never a real person. His existence is through "God" who is dead, through an inner world which is a persecutory system of internal bad objects fixated at the narcissistic stage. He is not interested in other men, nor in their liberation. When he finds he cannot be somebody, he wants to be a nobody, but compromises at being the leader of an army he does not want to lead. Goetz is who Sartre would like to be,[60] but from the start to the finish of the play, the same framework

53. Sartre, *The Devil and the Good Lord*, p. 147.
54. Ibid., p. 33.
55. Ibid., p. 137 ff.
56. Ibid., p. 146.
57. Ibid., p. 141.
58. Ibid., pp. 148-49.
59. Ibid., pp. 141, 149.
60. *See* Ch. 1.

remains for Goetz, except that he has rid himself of his illusions about doing Good and Evil to be noticed by a God he finds not to exist at all. The last Act puts Goetz back to the first, but without these illusions. He has recognized that the human world is the only one that exists and somewhat stoically defies the absence of God. There is no transformation of attitudes, merely a resignation to the facts of God's non-existence. Goetz is as much the bastard, abandoned and condemned to be of no account, yet still yearning for an absolute he now knows not to exist.

Goetz the evil, Goetz the good and Goetz the disillusioned "realist" maintain the same dramatic framework of inner and outer object-relations; it is just some of the objects that change. It is the same systemic torture house run on hate. He realizes he must show himself somehow that he exists, whether through God, through the hate of others or through his hate of himself. For Goetz it is hate or nothing. The inner system comprises persecutor and persecuted, torturer and victim, tempter and tempted, hater and hated; each internal object pitting its "freedom" against the others in a struggle which will only die with the death of Goetz himself. Goetz's power is power over himself; alone he is his only companion to whom he may demonstrate existence. He is not *de trop*: the torture situation, as has been argued above, can represent an ultimate and all-consuming sense of reality. For the torturer is taking great note of his victim—he wants to capture him and make his submission total. Yet the fight in Goetz is for what? Neither side can win or else there will be nothing—it is a static internal situation run on hate, but it is never fulfilling since this inner persecutory system is a defence against the feeling of being nothing at all. This is Goetz's constant feeling and fear which is only partly attenuated by the terrible reality of his inner world. Both the inner torturer and his victim go on because they are afraid of not doing so, afraid that the torture is not for anything at all and that the reality outside the torture house would be annihilating.

The paranoid who feels everyone is persecuting him is actually afraid that no one is taking any note of him whatever.[61] Sisyphus keeps pushing the boulder up the hill since there is nothing else he can do in the universe which imprisons him. The images of Goetz's inner world is for Sartre the image of the outer world too:[62] the political stage is set in a world in which meaning can come only through sado-masochistic relations for none other can exist. Transcendence — individual or social — towards a world in which we

61. Laing, *Self and Others*, p. 136.
62. de Beauvoir, *Force of Circumstance*, p. 254.

might be ontologically secure can never count as a possibility since after all we are nothing. After the revolution all we may do is contemplate our emptiness. In the world of allness or nothingness of power and impotence, autonomy in relations of "mature dependence"[63] just cannot get started except through our deceiving ourselves that we *are* something after all. Sartre's ontology, whether "existentialist" or "Marxist" precludes liberation at the same time as making it a necessity. Authentic reciprocity - one of Sartre's constant pre-occupations - has no ground from which to emerge: refusal is the highest form of being.

But Sartre has always been occupied with the position of the "third" perhaps because, partly conditioned by his own position, he was on the edge between the two great opposing forces; the working class and the bourgeoisie. Born a bourgeois, but rejecting the bourgeoisie, he was for the working class but not of it. He was a bastard through living the contradiction between his bourgeois birth and his intellectual choice.[64] The third who objectifies relationships by the possibility of his looking through the keyhole in *Being and Nothingness*, the third person in *Huis Clos* who destroys collusive possibilities; the third grouping which he among others set up in 1948[65], a socialist Europe as a third force to mediate between the USA and the USSR,[66] the third as potential mediator in the *Critique*[67], and most recently the fascination with "third" world struggles and politics. The third has a different position in a system from the antagonists—the third is on the edge, sometimes coming from outside. The third can be very powerful in destroying collusive relations as in *Huis Clos*, or it may be virtually powerless as the fellow-travelling "useless mouth" was to the P.C.F. in the 1940's.[68] Certainly politically, the third is in a rather powerless position because it is not a matter of demystifying or seeing through a situation so that it is thereby transformed; this is only the first step - the next is a matter of sheer power.

Sartre's relations with the P.C.F. revolve around the question of the viability of a third alternative to the bourgeois and the communist positions. The P.C.F. has been well-known for its extraordinarily doctrinaire authoritarian Stalinist position. Sartre's discussion of

63. Guntrip; *Personality Structure*, p. 357 ff.
64. de Beauvoir, *Force of Circumstance*, p. 253.
65. *Rassemblement Démocratique Révolutionnaire*. *See* Contat and Rybalka, pp. 199-205.
66. Sartre et al (1949), *Entretiens sur la politique*, pp. 185-86.
67. Sartre, *Critique de la raison dialectique*, pp. 753-54.
68. Sartre, *What is Literature?*, p. 191 ff.

Marxism is strangely contemporary with the attitude of the P.C.F. The early Marx seems not to have been discovered by Sartre until the 1960s: in *Search for a Method* he quotes a statement by Engels as representing "the" Marxist position.[69] There has never been a question of Sartre and the R.C.F. going their independent ways while ignoring each other. Sartre's stress on the importance of the P.C.F. is understandable since the C.P.'s in France and Italy—as opposed to those in other Western countries—are the major mass party and command the support of a large section of the proletariat.[70]

The peculiar position that the P.C.F. has always occupied in French politics cannot be overstressed. Its tyrannical, monolithic, hierarchical Stalinist structure predominates over any oppositional or independent positions. Very little influence is exercised by the "soldiers of the party" in the lower levels—decisions are made at the top and relayed downward to the rank and file who carry out the instructions and politics. Its very close ties with the working class make the P.C.F. the exclusively "effective" political agent of social change, and to be divorced from the P.C.F. is to live in a political wasteland for people on the left. The problems Sartre describes which relate to the choice between a religious adherence to the quasi-divine and all-powerful party machine and individual freedom must be seen as very real in this light. The P.C.F. has always lived and created a world of its own: the Party has always been the *corpus mysticum*, and a commitment to it meant loss of an individual identity while to be outside of it meant living in a political desert very far from the proletariat who see the P.C.F. as their representative.

Sartre himself has been subject to the most scurrilous attacks by P.C.F. spokesmen who have denounced him as a "cop-intellectual", a "philosopher of the graveyard", "an understudy of Koestler". Garaudy wrote in 1947: "Every class has the literature it deserves. The big bourgeoisie in decay delights in the obsessions of Henry Miller or the fornications of Jean-Paul Sartre". Sartre was described in the Soviet press as "the servile executor of a mission confided in him by Wall Street".[71] Garaudy wrote in a book denouncing existentialism that it was "sick" and that the theses of *Being and Nothingness* remain in the realm of "metaphysical pathology".[72] At other times the P.C.F. has forgotten its past difference with Sartre -

69. Sartre, *Search for a Method*, Ch. 1.
70. R. Aron, *The Opium of the Intellectuals*, p. 157.
71. D. Caute, *The Fellow Travellers: A Postscript to the Enlightment*, p. 346.
72. R. Garaudy, "False Prophet: Jean-Paul Sartre" in G. Novack (ed.), *Existentialism versus Marxism: Conflicting Views on Humanism*, p. 156.

as Sartre has with it—and has acclaimed him at various times.[73]

Since the war Sartre has been a most important figure in France, a celebrity as well as a scandal to both the bourgeoisie and the P.C.F. He raised the questions people were asking even though his answers may not have been to their liking.[74] The publicity, passions and intensity given to debates such as those between Sartre and Camus or Merleau-Ponty are immensely greater than similar ones would be in other countries. Aron wonders why "French intellectuals, whether Christians, Socialists, Guallists, Communists or Existentialists vie with one another in talk of Revolution".[75] Perhaps this atmosphere contributed to the importance Sartre gave the P.C.F. However, this does not account for Sartre taking the P.C.F. as representing Marxism since he was aware of other "Marxisms"—e.g. he held the Italian C.P. in very high regard.[76] Probably however, this strange fact mirrors how strongly Sartre sees the binary constitution of politics.

Ultimately, politically one was either for or against the Party if no "third force" seemed viable. In this situation if a person was against the Party, this meant objectively that he lined himself up with the capitalists: thus the problems about whether Sartre ought to denounce the Soviet Labour Camps.[77] The Kafkaesque world the intellectual encountered in the P.C.F. was baldly denounced by Sartre in 1947,[78] and never retracted afterward, even where a "third" force was not a possibility. It was a primary duty of the writer to write freely, and this would in fact best help the cause.[79] But even after the Soviet intervention in Hungary which he unreservedly condemned, calling *L'Humanité*'s reports "repugnant lies",[80] he wrote that his aim had always been the same in violence and in friendship with the C.P.: to promote a unity of all the left-wing parties which alone could save France. But to join with the C.P. as it was then "would be to compromise the last chances of a single front"—but the main task of intellectuals was not to put forward an independent view to the masses, but "to try to help in the de-stalinization of the French Party".[81]

73. Caute, *The Fellow Travellers*, p. 344 ff.
74. de Beauvoir, *force of Circumstance*, pp.47-48.
75. Aron, *The Opium of the Intellectuals*, pp. 57-58.
76. Sartre has even said (to Burnier): "If I were in Italy, I would join the Party". Burnier, *Choice of Action*, p. 140.
77. Sartre, *Reply to Albert Camus*, passim. de Beauvoir, *Force of Circumstance*, p. 209 ff.
78. Sartre, *What is Literature?*, p. 191.
79. Ibid., pp. 210-12.
80. Caute, *Communism and the French Intellectuals*, p. 255.
81. Sartre (1956-57), *The Spectre of Stalin*, p. 108.

The formation of the R.D.R. as a third movement took place in an atmosphere in which it was possible to see the Marshall Plan as trying to create a bulwark against Russia, but which could be used peacefully and effectively if controlled by European Socialism.[82] This was an unusual situation in which the position of the post-war antagonists would be used to the advantage of the French revolutionaries. Europe need not pass through Soviet-style communism to achieve socialism.[83] But this turned out to be unworkable and his love-hate relations with the P.C.F. became dominant once again. Jeanson divides his attitude to the P.C.F. into four phases:—a resolutely critical attitude from 1945 to 1950, rapprochement from 1951 to 1956; from Hungary 1956 to the end of the Algerian War in 1962 a sharpening of differences; and from 1962 a new but critical rapprochement.[84] A fifth period may now be added: from the 1968 events in France (and Czechoslovakia) to the present, Sartre has become very critical indeed of the P.C.F. and takes an independent "maoist"-style position.[85] So at least until around 1968 his political point of reference and axis around which to revolve, was basically the P.C.F. The question of whether or not to join the Party was a major one in the 1940s and 1950s as is shown in Sartre's own work, particularly in the Mathieu-Brunet interactions, and in de Beauvoir's books, especially *The Blood of Others*. The Party represented the second against the first world and Sartre and his colleagues played a more or less feeble third.

But what about the established order being attacked? Before the war, Sartre had not voted and felt outside politics. If anything, he reflected the anarchist sympathies of his generation.[86] During the war, Sartre decided he would go into politics and actively fought for a third in a left-of-centre France. With the deepening of the Cold War and the Korean War, he became very involved in anti-American and anti-government activity culminating in *The Communists and Peace*. About the execution of the Rosenbergs, Sartre wrote that America was "in the cradle of a new fascism... for fascism is not defined by the number of its victims, but by the way it kills them".[87] He later became very involved on the extreme left in the Algerian War, which instituted a growing interest in the third

82. Sartre et al, *Entretiens sur la politique*, pp. 85-86. Caute, *Communism and the French Intellectuals*, p. 250. Burnier, *Choice of Action*, p. 32.
83. Sartre et al, Idem.
84. Jeanson, *Sartre par lui-même*, pp. 117-18.
85. Sartre, "On Maoism". Interview with Contat, *Le Nouvel Observateur*.
86. de Beauvoir, *The Prime of Life*, p. 169.
87. Cited and translated in Caute, *Communism and the French Intellectuals*, p. 254.

world as the first and second worlds drew toward a greater integration within their own countries and between them. The attitudes of the P.C.F. to the "Algerian problem" highlighted for Sartre how integrated the working class had become. This integration is reflected strongly in the *Critique*. His travels in South America, Cuba and China, the Vietnam War and the Russell War Crimes Tribunal, sharpened his identification with the wretched of the earth confronted with imperialist brutality. Like his maoist comrades, he refuses to work within the system, and again does not even vote for that would imply an acceptance of its institutions.

> How can legal action—the Communist Party's for example—overthrow the law? It will necessarily destroy itself in contortions so absurd as to be improbably. This is one reason I am drawn to the Maoists: I believe in illegality.[88]

Besides the P.C.F., representing the Communist bloc, the other relatively constant axis of reference Sartre took seriously was the U.S.A. America had always fascinated Sartre, and apart from his travels there, he has written much about it. He has written essays on American cities, pointing to their vastness and openness, essays eulogizing das Passos and Faulkner, numerous articles, a play, *The Respectful Prostitute*, and many political commentaries.[89] The USA is the only first world country, other than France, that receives attention besides being the mere setting of a play. *Altona* was prompted by the Algerian War;[90] *The Devil and the Good Lord* is an epic far more of the past than of another country; *Les Mains sales* is set in Illyria, which de Beauvoir informs us was inspired by Hungary,[91] but even here it is more concerned with the problem raised by a revolutionary situation, one which France had never encountered. For the rest, Sartre mainly writes about France, and most of his political writings where they discuss events in other countries, relate back to the problems of the left in France.[92] The exceptions to this seem to be his writings about the third world.[93] Much reference has

88. Sartre, "On Maoism", p. 101.
89. Sartre (1945), "American Cities" in *Literary and Philosophical Essays*. Sartre (1945), "Individualism and Conformism in the United States" in ibid. Sartre (1946), "New York, the Colonial City" in ibid. Sartre (1946), "American Novelists in French Eyes", *Atlantic Monthly*. Sartre (1946), *The Respectful Prostitute*. Sartre (1947), "Americans and Their Myths", *Nation* CLXV. Sartre (1965), "Why I will Not Go to the United States", *Nation* CC.
90. Sartre (1961), "An Interview with Jean-Paul Sartre", *The Tullane Drama Review* V, pp. 13-14.
91. de Beauvoir; *Force of Circumstance*, p. 162.
92. Sartre; *The Spectre of Stalin*.
93. For example, Sartre (1960), *Sartre on Cuba*.

been made to Sartre's "anti-Americanism",[94] but less note seems to have been taken of the near love-hate relationship he seems to have with it.

The intensity of his feeling about America can be seen in the statement about fascism quoted above together with the defiant statement that "we will *never* give leadership of the Western World to the murderers of the Rosenbergs". And most revealingly:

> Do not be surprised if we shout from one end of Europe to the other, "Beware, America has the rabies. Let us cut the bonds that bind us to her; otherwise we will in our turn be bitten and infected".[95]

America had stood for harshness, pragmatism, and was the homeland of capitalism, It had been the centre of the world and its supreme power.[96] Everything is provisional and temporary. The cities of America are open, "open to the world and to the future. This gives them their adventurous look, and even in their ugliness and disorder, a touching beauty".[97] Sartre was fascinated with the degree to which American myths contrasted with their reality.

I could amplify this evidence for Sartre's near-obsession with America as the most powerful, vicious, new, complex and fascinating nation which somehow defied definition.[98] But one incident in particular exemplifies his attitude well. Sartre had agreed to deliver a series of lectures at Cornell in 1965, and cancelled them. He said that he would not go to the US while it was committing the atrocities in Vietnam. The Americans seemed as mystified about Vietnam as were the French with Algeria. There was no possibility of dialogue with the Americans, only a small number of whom would take any notice of him anyway. The political weight of the Americans who were against the Vietnam war was unhappily "nil". The opponents of the Vietnam War in America formed only a tiny minority of intellectuals and were "totally impotent". The man on the American Left who saw through the almost all-pervasive myths of imperialism and anti-communism was, Sartre says, "indeed one of the accursed of the earth. He totally disapproves of the politics carried out in his name and his action is totally ineffective—in any case, for the present". Sartre's characteristic alternative of "all or nothing" could not be

94. For example, Caute, *Communism and the French Intellectuals*, p. 253. Cranston, "Sartre and Violence", p. 19.
95. Cited and translated in Burnier, *Choice of Action*, pp. 98-99.
96. Sartre, "Why I Will Not Go to the United States", p. 411.
97. Sartre, "American Cities", p. 117.
98. Sartre, "New York, the Colonial City", p. 118.

clearer. He even identifies the perceptive American intellectual as on the same basis as he does the third world revolutionaries: America however seems done for: Sartre is disillusioned with this country which had seemed to hold out certain possibilities for an open future and in his disappointment, he refused to even go there. The following passage deserves quoting at length:

> I wish to say, also, that we do not now have to regard America as the center of the world. It is the greatest power in the world? Granted. But note: it is far from being the center of it. When one is European, one has the duty even not to consider America as the world's center; one has to show one's interest in and prove one's solidarity with the people of Vietnam, Cuba, and Africa with all one's friends in the "third world" who have thrust themselves to the threshold of existence and of freedom, and who prove each day that the greatest power in the world is incapable of imposing its laws, that it is also the most vulnerable power in the world, and that the world has not chosen it to be its center of gravity. The United States will evolve slowly, very slowly. And more, I think if one resists it, than if one preaches to it.[99]

Sartre quite obviously believes that America *is* the centre of gravity in the world—he admits that he *had* thought it was, and that Europeans should now shift their focus on to the struggles in the third world. But against whom are the third world battling? America. So we have the typical Sartrean torture situation—a mighty torturer trying to control a seemingly powerless victim without resources. The torturer has reduced all opposition inside him to impotence, and presents a univocal evil with highly sophisticated instruments of torture and death. The opposition within is truly accursed, and can be saved only by the third world comrades the US moloch is taking on. Is this perhaps like the French during the Algerian War or under the German Occupation? What can the intellectual do standing on the sidelines—except write? America is the enemy to be beaten. What Sartre is really saying is that we should see as a myth the view that America is the strongest power and cannot be fought with any degree of success at all—as Henri Alleg had shown in the Algerian war. If America is not the central power, it is part of the central struggle. It is unequivocally on the most powerful yet at the same time most wrong side—not an unusual position for Sartre to assume. The power-impotence relationship instantiates itself once again as primary; it is possible to win, but not from within.

In point of fact, Sartre had misread the situation. The editors of

99. Sartre, "Why I Will Not Go to the United States", pp. 408-11.

*The Nation* pointed out that it was precisely because resistance from within was significant that Sartre's support was requested in the first place.[100]

Sartre must have recognized his error for the teach-in group at Boston University received a cable from Sartre in contrast with his earlier scornful dismissal of American academics:

> I am sorry that I cannot be present with you today (sic!) but I want you to know that I am in complete sympathy with your demonstration. It is comforting for us to see that the opposition of the intellectuals grows stronger every day. (And still more interestingly, the demonstrations) take place at a moment when irresponsible men are engaged in presenting to the world an odious image of your country and they will help them to realize *that this image is false, and that the rising generation is determined to dissociate itself from it completely.*

Moreover he sees "every reason to hope" that there will be a "profound change" in the U.S.A. and in the world when the youth come of age.[101] The image of the irresponsible men in control of the USA created three weeks before was then completely true—now it is completely false. Where three weeks before he would not even set foot on US soil, he now "regrets" not being able to attend a teach-in in which the intellectuals he had scorned and pitied would take part. Perhaps the image of a pure and idealistic rising generation played a part in his *volte face*. But what is obvious is the extremism of his views— all or nothing, the new generation will crush the old. As Simone de Beavoir has remarked in another connection, Sartre never resorts to half measures.[102] The point being made is not a psychologically reductionist one; in fact the seemingly almighty powers of the US regime have taken a beating both from within the US and from outside it in the valiant, determined and successful struggle of the Vietnamese people. But this point remains in the events described: Sartre's attitude towards a very significant America is one of idealization (certainly not simply of idealism) to which the facts seem to provide a backdrop. Sartre is not "anti-American" as he has himself stated:[103] he is quite ambivalent towards it. As he wrote of America as early as 1947, "Perhaps nowhere else will you find such a discrepancy between people and myth, between life and the represen-

100. *Nation* editorial, "On the Need for Dialogue", p. 408.
101. Sartre (1965), Cable cited in "Up All Night", *Nation* CC, p. 574. (My emphasis.)
102. "Sartre never stopped halfway in any enterprise..." de Beauvoir, *The Prime of Life*, p. 288. Cranston, "Sartre and Violence, p. 19.
103. Sartre (1946); Letter in *New York Herald Tribune*, (European Edition).

tation of life".[104] But which is myth and which is reality sometimes seems unclear to Sartre. What is clear is that America the tyrant, the monster or the resurgent, pure, open future, is powerful, fascinating and real to Sartre. The opposition within or without will recognize itself in its relations of conflict with American power. At the same time, however, America may not be so bad after all — the true America may yet show itself true to its myths or to its reality whatever these may be. Sartre very much makes a stand, perhaps as a witness.

His refusal to go to the US followed a refusal to accept the Nobel Prize for Literature in the previous year. This peculiar incident is again typically Sartrean and illustrates Sartre's primary process thinking remarkably well. As ever Sartre the writer does not want to be institutionalized and wants his works to be read as written simply by Jean-Paul Sartre, not Jean-Paul Sartre the Nobel Prize laureate. Of course, ironically the only man of the century to refuse the Nobel Prize, he will be the more avidly read as Jean-Paul Sartre—the man who refused the Nobel Prize. Sartre even maintained:[105]

> My sympathies for the Venezuelan revolutionists commit only myself, while Jean-Paul Sartre the Nobel laureate champions the Venezuelan resistance, he also commits the entire Nobel Prize as an institution.

This logic is patently absurd, but if maintained would militate against the "objective reasons" he professes for his refusing the Prize. The Nobel Prize, he maintains, stands objectively as a distinction reserved for writers of the West or rebels of the East, and is thus a political rather than a literary one. If it had been awarded him during the Algerian hostilities, he would gladly have accepted it "because it would have honoured not only me, but also the freedom for which we were fighting". He wonders why it is only "after the battle is over that the prize has been awarded me". So it had been denied him on political grounds, but he would then have *accepted* it on political grounds. But the prize should be given on *literary* grounds and not institutionalize the writer in any way, no matter how beneficial to a cause it may be. Nor should the writer chain the institution to a political cause such as the Venezuelan guerrillas with whom he sympathises!

But there are further contradictory turns: freedom, Sartre declares, is more concrete than the general freedom meant in the West. This concrete freedom "consists of the right to have more than

104. Sartre. "Americans and their Myths", p. 403.
105. Sartre, "Sartre and the Nobel Prize".

one pair of shoes and to eat one's fill". If that is so, he should be pleased to accept the Prize and donate the money to the Anti-Apartheid Movement—which he would have done, had he accepted the Prize. This would have helped that Movement which badly needed financial support, as Sartre acknowledged... "But", he adds, "one cannot be asked to renounce for 250,000 crowns principles which are not only one's own, but are shared by his comrades". Sartre is here using the old "Western" version of freedom he renounces to prevail over the concrete freedom he here advocates!

There are still more contradictions which need not detain us in this extraordinary "explanation" for Sartre's refusal of the Nobel Prize. His position is absurd on a rational level. But it well demonstrates some of his own conflicts and confusions in the form of rationalization.[106] These conflicts are not only Sartre's, as he himself would be the first to proclaim, but some of the conflicts of our time. But in fact, as one observer put it: "Sartre's renunciation sprang from an impulsive need to stay on the good side of his own conscience, and not at all as he pretends, on the inexorable logic of the committed writer". Sartre had rejected the Nobel Prize "to keep his hands clean" and "not to bear witness to the responsibility of the writer of modern times".[107] I shall return to the aspect of clean versus dirty hands in due course for this is not Sartre's problem alone: it reflects the complexities of modern living. But before doing so through "sociological" concepts, I want to refer to some "psycho-social" categories.

In his *Psychopathology and Politics* Laswell had written that politics was the only area of public life in which people were expected to act rationally. In fact, however, there was often a displacement of private motives into the public arena. However, the "private" motives not only condition but at least as importantly are conditioned by the social milieux—there is a dialectical relationship between them, and a study of "private" depths casts much light on the age itself—an age which conditions the neurotic personality of our time. Indeed Sartre has always been interested in the relationship between "public" and "private" affairs among people involved in politics.

The student of Sartre and Laswell may well be struck by the ap-

106. This is not to say that there could not be an argument for refusing the Prize. Nor is it to deny the very deep affinity Sartre has with revolutionary struggles.
107. N. Chiaromonte, "Sartre and the Prize", *Encounter* XXII, p. 57.

plicability of Laswell's agitator-theorist categories to Sartre. However, this ought not to be too surprising since both Laswell and Sartre are mediated by, and are part of the era they live and study. Sartre is, of course, both an agitator and a theorist, sometimes one rather than the other predominating. But Laswell notes the interrelations of agitators and theorists, remarking that it is "often simply a matter of taste whether emphasis is to be placed on one or other feature of the history". Laswell's theorists have characteristically sought to influence their contemporaries.[108] Indeed Sartre's "committed literature" provides a perfect bridge here between theorist and agitator. Laswell's formulation deserves quotation at length.

> Agitators as a class are strongly narcissistic types. Narcissism is encouraged by obstacles in the early love relationships, or by overindulgence and admiration in the family circle. Libido which is blocked in moving outward toward objects settles back upon the self. Sexual objects like the self are preferred, and a strong homosexual component is thus characteristic. Among the agitators this yearning for emotional response of the homosexual kind is displaced upon generalized objects, and high value is placed on arousing emotional responses from the community at large. The tremendous urge for expression in written or spoken language is a roundabout method of gratifying these underlying emotional drives. Agitators show many traits which are characteristic of primitive narcissism in the exaggerated value which they put on the efficacy of formulas and gestures in producing results in the world of objective reality. The family history shows much repression of the direct manifestation of hatred. There is often a record of a "model boy" during the early years, of a shy and sensitive child who swallowed his resentments. Repressed sadism is partly vented upon objects remote from the immediately given environment and favours the cultivation of general social interests. The youth has usually learned to control by suppression and by repression the full amplitude of his affects - this is a discipline in deceit. The narcissistic reactions prevent the developing individual from entering into full and warm emotional relationships... They show marked predominance of oral traits.
>
> Those consciously attached to their parents... and who have been successful impostors, are disposed to choose remote and general objects... the rational structure tends toward theoretical completeness. Displacement choices depend on the models available, when early identifications are made... When the homosexual attitude is particularly important, the assaultive provocative relation to the environment is likely to develop itself; when the impotence fear is active, grandiose reaction patterns appear more prominently.[109]

108. H. Laswell, *Psychopathology and Politics*, p. 54.
109. Ibid., pp. 125-26. *See also* p.262.

Sartre is the model child and impostor who has compulsive urges to express himself and his world orally; who systematizes at a highly abstract level, while at the same time actively attacking all in any type of authority; who depicts all relationships as mutually devouring. The best relationships in Sartre's work are generally between men, such as Brunet and Vicarios in *La Dernière chance*, Hugo and Hoederer in *Les Mains sales*, between men and the quasi-religious organization of the P.C.F., or the religious zeal of a committed literature. Women fare very badly indeed in Sartre's world—they are gross, small-minded, ugly, selfish, manipulative and try to prevent their men taking action.[110] Impotence is a major theme for Sartre—the power principle prevailing easily over any pleasure principle whatever: sex is almost always odious in Sartre's work. The fight for control is, of course, more primitive than mature sexuality which presupposes quite a degree of autonomy. Sartre himself admits in *Words* to having been victim to all kinds of illusions, not the least of which was the projection of an ontology on to the world scene which represented his own state of being (as well as that of many others). The past scarcely figures in Sartre's early work, and he himself remarks how he used not to recognize that he even had a childhood.[111] Sartre had obviously repressed it, displacing his affects on to grand political and theoretical planes.

Laswell observes that "the unconscious hatred of authority discloses itself in the endless capacity of the theorist to imagine new reasons for disbelieving and in his capacity to labour over the trivialities and reduce his whole intellectual scheme to logical absurdity. Words lose their rational reference points and become packed with unconscious symbolism of the ambivalent variety".[112] This should be abundantly obvious in Sartre who seems a paradigm case here. Doubts about himself have been displaced on to the world outside—and he attempts to allay these doubts by what Laswell terms "ostentatious pre-occupation with the truth". Sartre who has always seen conflict as the major form of relationship exemplifies Laswell's dictum that "there is little boldness in political thinking which is not accompanied by an overdose of defiance".[113]

It should be stressed again that I am not trying to reduce Sartre's work psychologistically, but attempting to reach a greater understanding of his work through the conditioning processes which themselves are exemplified in it. On one level we may ask whether a

110. Lilar, *A propos de Sartre et de l'amour*, Ch. 4.
111. Sartre, *Words*, p. 148.
112. Laswell, *Psychopathology and Politics*, p. 175.
113. Ibid., pp. 175-76.

particular attitude is correct. But this by no means excludes a dialectical, biographical approach which includes this question among others which deal with the context in which the question arises. That Sartre exemplifies Laswell's agitator-theorist paradigmatically does not mean that Sartre's work is therefore of little importance. On the contrary, it shows itself as being of immense importance if only because its expression is a lucid embodiment of the contemporary human scene. He expresses the scene and reactions to it; the range of alternatives and goals that appear realistic and desirable, and the general social context, with its influences from micro-social to macro-social events. Thus there is normally an over-determination of causes; and it is in an understanding of these that a more total comprehension of the person in his situation may be grounded.

In a book devoted to the "communist problem" written during the McCarthy era, Almond has some interesting observations about "types of neurotic susceptibility" to communism.[114] Even here, there is no attempt to explain the appeal communist party membership has for certain people **solely** in terms of psychological factors. Almond, who uses a medical model of communism as a disease, points to psychological factors which might *predispose* people to enter the C.P. rather than *causing* them to do so.

The kind of person he describes as having "neurotic susceptibility" is remarkably like the agitator-theorist models of Laswell. Feelings of inferiority, of unworthiness, of emptiness and withdrawness, of self-rejection and isolation, of fear, repression and displacement of hostility, fear of abandonment, represented prominent patterns in people who were attracted to the Party. The Party may represent an image of salvation for such alienated and rootless people. The C.P. may offer everything to the person who feels he has nothing, and has more or less unconscious hostility towards his surroundings. The Party represents not only a community, but a hostile community for outcasts.[115] The description that Almond gives "of some of the sorts of people attracted to the Party", adequately fits the "intellectual bastards" Sartre describes. The Party offers these people everything they have missed out on and crave in the Marxist classics and in the communist media of communication. There is constant emphasis on organization, community, relatedness. The ideal image of the communist conveys the impression of a man who has his place in the meaningful progression of time, and who is surrounded by steadfast and loyal comrades. The communist militant is not only

114. G.A. Almond, *The Appeals of Communism*, Ch. 10.
115. Ibid., p. 270.

related to a group; he also shares in a kind of mystical body, he merges himself in the *corpus mysticum* of the party, acquires a larger identity from it, and even a sense of "immortality".[116] Further the image of the communist militant is of a "dignified, special person, dedicated, strong, confident of the future, a man who knows his objectives, does his duty without hesitation".[117]

The description Almond gives is the one Sartre gives of Brunet of the P.C.F. in *The Roads to Freedom*. And the attraction to this is seen by Mathieu who represents the person in great need of it.[118] The "mystical body" certainly accurately represents the P.C.F. The alternatives that Sartre gives were the only possible ones in the France he describes: the rootless alienation of the abandoned intellectual who feels unreal and more dead than alive, and the solid soldier of the Party who knows where he is going and has a strong sense of being alive, even though it is through the mystical body of the Party and the USSR. The third alternative of a responsible man of action who is independent, autonomous and spontaneous in his interactions never even arises for Sartre in an all or nothing, power or impotence situation. The actual world seemed to posit these alternatives exclusively, and it is Sartre's vain and impotent efforts to find a third way between the solid and monstrous forces of reaction and the Party that raise the question of the feasibility of individuality in the contemporary world. The alienated intellectual is faced with a given situation of two opposing forces, allegiance to either of which means engulfment and loss of self. But without being at home with one of these gargantuan monsters, the intellectual has nothing whatever. Brunet could dismiss introspective comments as "psychological balderdash",[119] and whenever a difficult situation arose, he could think of the Party and feel safe and certain. On the other hand, Mathieu could see the benefits of such a womb-like situation, but also the self-deceiving loss of individuality involved.

To dismiss Sartre's reactions as pathological entirely misses the point that the reality he faced was actually like that - Sartre's schizoid despair reflects the schizoid character of the culture he lived. His image of the P.C.F. was one which was unhappily realistic, as was his description of the anomic bourgeois who rejected the bourgeoisie but was not accepted by the other great force - the

116. Ibid., p. 272.
117. Ibid., p. 279.
118. *See* Ch. 2.
119. "The iron in the soul — all right, but what then? 'Just a lot of psychological balderdash', he [Brunet] said to himself scornfully. He came to a stop, thinking of the Party". Sartre, *Iron in the Soul*, p. 316.

Party of the working class. He is between two worlds, having no identity in either. He realizes his plight but is powerless to do anything about it. The individual is alone in confronting a world consisting not of individuals, but of anonymously powerful forces which seem to have absorbed the people who are part of them. The outsider can see but he cannot act effectively. The person who is part of the Party, who sees only through its machine, may act "effectively", but not in his own terms as a person for the "Cause", since the direction is prescribed from outside. For Sartre, the world seems a mass of contradictory forces in which intentions and actions, individuality and autonomous power seem irrevocably divorced, distorted and dislocated. A sense of belonging is a sham in such a world since actions and their consequences do not appear to belong to men, but men seem appendages to their roles in a topsy turvy world of radical alienation.

In this alienated world, what are the real possibilities of revolutionary political action which will help bring about human liberation? What can be done? Sartre sees two choices generally: to become part of the C.P. and abdicate general principles in favour of the furthering of the "Cause" no matter what the cost; or to always stand by the principles for which one is fighting under all circumstances - truth, justice, honesty: hands covered with blood or purity and cleanliness? Is the good action the "effective" one or the "principled" one? It may be maintained that the best action is the one which is both principled and effective, but what about the normal situations where there seems to be a contradiction? In the best of all possible worlds, there may not be a contradiction of ends and means, for the good end is embodied in means that will harm no one.

But what of the world today? Sartre is well aware of this problem. Goetz, in his attempt to do good, in fact does irreparable harm to the cause of the peasants. "In one day of virtue, you killed more people than in thirty-five years of malice", Heinrich tells Goetz the saint.[120] Violence is sometimes not only justified but necessary. Suppression of certain freedoms is sometimes seen as necessary for the sake of the preservation or attainment of others. Accordine to Sartre, "We must begin by realizing that we live in a violent world, that violence was not invented by those who are now using it: that all is violence". The writer must construct his own theory of violence and understand "that there is violence to fight violence".[121] He must not condemn violence *a priori*, but must condemn only "useless violence".

120. Sartre, *The Devil and the Good Lord*, p. 138.
121. Sartre, "The Responsibility of the Writer", p. 81.

Violence must be understood in its setting and not in the abstract.[122] We cannot stand by abstract principles which, if implemented, would in fact bring great harm. The realization of certain principles for which revolutionaries have been fighting might well bring about the downfall of the revolutionary state itself as in *L'Engrenage*. If men are defined by their actions, and the consequences of them, then someone with the best will and principles in the world may be defined as being objectively a social fascist or class traitor. But we have seen that in the world Sartre describes there is a paradoxical effect of actions - loser wins. If this is the case, then we might sometimes lie for the sake of truth—certainly we should "play politics".

However, as I have argued the playing of politics is overdetermined. Why did Hugo kill Hoederer? For private or public motives? Because no matter what his intentions, Hoederer was an objective traitor? Because Hoederer had tricked him into trusting him? Because Hugo saw that all along Hoederer was only interested in an affair with Jessica? Because the assassination would serve the interest of the Party of the working class? So that Hugo might have a sense of belonging, of reality? There are so many interwoven reasons the unthreading of which is very difficult, but one very real conflict is clear: that of purity versus soiled hands, of principle versus effectiveness and responsibility, of idealism versus realism.

Hugo incarnates the intellectual idealist who joins the Party ostensibly because its cause is just.[123] There is never more than one end: "to put into practice our ideals, all our ideals and nothing but our ideals".[124] He cannot countenance Hoederer's negotiating with the fascist Regent whom they had been fighting and lying to his comrades. For Hugo at home everyone had lied to himself, and to him also. When he joined the Party, Hugo found himself in a situation in which nobody lied to himself or others, and everybody could trust everyone else. "The most unimportant member felt that the orders of the leaders revealed to him his deepest desire and that if there was a difficult job to be done, one knew why one agreed to die". For Hugo, the only good methods are ones derived from principle - lying for example can never be excused. On the other hand, Hoederer believes the good method to be the effective one.[125] He lies when he must, but despises no one. His hands are soiled with blood. It is impossible "to govern and keep your spirit white".[126] A certain compromise of prin-

122. Ibid., p. 82.
123. Sartre, *Crime Passionnel*, p. 96.
124. Ibid., p. 93.
125. Ibid., p. 94.
126. Ibid., p. 95.

ciples might mean saving hundreds of thousands of lives which Hugo would be prepared to sacrifice for the sake of his principles. According to Hoederer, Hugo does not love his fellow man, but rather his principles. Hugo replies:

> As for my fellow men, it isn't what they *are* that interests me, but what they may become.
>
> **Hoederer:** And I love them for what they are. With all their squalors and all their vices, I love their voices and their warm hands, their worried looks and their desperate struggle against death and unhappiness. For me, a man more or less in the world, that's important. His life is precious. I know you, my boy, you're a destroyer. You hate men because you hate yourself; your purity is the purity of death and the revolution you dream of isn't ours; you don't want to change the world, you want to blow it apart.[127]

The man who lives for idealistic principles is then not interested in *real* men and situations, but *ideal* men and situations—ideal because he despises or cannot contact the real world. The man who stands by his principles does not feel responsible for the consequences of his actions. The man of principles lives in his own world even—perhaps especially—when he carries out political action. While idealism ought to represent the realization of ideals, there is no straight and easy path to such realization in the real world—in contrast to the phantasy world of the idealist. The idealist may be caught in the net of idealization of the state of the world and his principles. Hugo treats men as means towards his ideal rather than as ends in themselves. Thus he would be prepared to sacrifice them for the sake of the principle of revolution, of truth. However, he does not take responsibility for this implication.

Hoederer on the other hand is aware of the practical consequence of his actions in the real world. He realizes that the world does not live up to our ideals of it, and that abstract idealistic principles may be destructive if implemented. Hoederer recognizes that acts are not intrinsically good or bad since their consequences may be bad or good, As opposed to Hugo, Hoederer is prepared to take responsibility for the consequences of his actions and not hide behind a screen of ideals, especially where these ideals betray a hatred of men as they are.

A similar situation is depicted in *L'Engrenage*. Jean the revolutionary leader who had taken power in a small country, Illyria, bordering a powerful country with large oil interests in Illyria, sup-

127. Ibid., p. 96.

presses democracy and discussion of the nationalization of oil. This he does because if he were to allow Illyrian people to do what they wanted and nationalize the oil industry, the neighbouring power would invade Illyria and crush the Revolution. Jean even sends his best friend, Lucien, an idealistic writer, to prison because Lucien was about to publish an article attacking Jean and calling for the nationalization of oil. Jean had asked Lucien why he wrote such articles. Lucien replied:

> "Because I think they're just".
>
> "It's too early - too early".
>
> "It's never too early to speak the truth... I've trusted you, Jean. Everybody's trusted you. But today we no longer understand you. You haven't nationalized oil. You haven't had a parliament elected. The press isn't free. It was for all that that we brought about the revolution".
>
> "If they elect a parliament", says Jean, "the first law they will pass will be the nationalization of oil".
>
> "That's what the whole country wants... Why don't you do it?"
>
> "We should be in danger of war. It's too early".[128]

Jean is prepared to go against the wishes of the country to save the revolution. Lucien wants his principles adhered to which would bring about the actual destruction of the revolution. Lucien, like Hugo, is more in love with his principles than with men.

In *Les Mains sales* Hoederer is shot; but ironically his approach is finally implemented by the Party. In *L'Engrenage*, Jean the tyrant is overthrown by his people; but there is only a change in personnel, not of policy. The new leader François receives a friendly call from the ambassador of the neighbouring country who threatens intervention if his country's oil interests are nationalized. François agrees not to interfere with the oil: *Plus ça change, plus c'est là même chose.*

It is difficult to face reality when it is so distant from our ideals. Max Weber was aware that the "fate of our times" was characterized above all by the "disenchantment of the world".[129] Indeed summer's bloom did not lie ahead but rather "a polar night of icy darkness and hardness, no matter which group may triumph externally now".[130] It takes great courage to face action in such a world. There are two ethics to which we may have recourse in politics: the "ethic of respon-

128. Sartre (1948), *In the Mesh, (L'Engrenage)*, p. 89.
129. M. Weber, "Science as a Vocation" in Gerth and Mills, p. 155.
130. M. Weber, "Politics as a Vocation" in Gerth and Mills, p. 128. Cf. Sartre's reference to "the great polar night of the inhuman", *What is Literature?*, p. 163.

sibility" and the "ethic of ultimate ends".[131] The latter incarnated in the attitude of Lucien and Hugo rests on the formula, "The world is stupid and base, not I", is not moved by any form of responsibility for the consequences of action. However, the "mature man" accepts the ethic of responsibility and really feels the responsibility for his actions "with his heart and soul", and reaches the point where he says, "Here I stand. I can do no other". For Weber, this is "genuinely human and moving" and relies on a sober assessment of the real situation, not an idealized one; on the assumption of responsibility for his acts and the consequences he foresees, rather than on abstract principles that belong to no one, but on which one can unload the burden.[132]

Weber delineates the domain of "legitimate violence" as the locus of the ethical problems in politics.[133] The man like Hoederer or Jean who accepts an "ethic of responsibility" accepts the average deficiencies of people, the necessities of violence of some form in politics, and does not ascribe the bad consequences of his actions to the stupidity or baseness of others or of the world itself.[134] Indeed, he claims his actions as his own. Principles such as truthfulness do not hold unconditionally as they do with the others of absolute ends which by their very nature can never ask for consequences. He can accept the paradoxical relation of action and its consequences, and can acknowledge this tragedy without recourse to self-deception or myths. An ethic of responsibility is an essential element of calling for politics as a vocation. He must be sure that he shall not crumble when the world seems too stupid or too base for what he wants to offer. Only he who in the face of all this can say "In spite of all!" has the calling for politics.[135] Hugo cannot do this, nor can Lucien. Yet Hoederer and Jean are obviously able to bear with the crumbling of their hopes. It is not that they do not hope and have lost their ideals, but rather that they have accommodated to realistic perspectives for amelioration. This need not—does not—imply conformity with the prevailing system—a reformism. This would be too easy since this would in fact imply the view that "the world is stupid and base, not I", that it is impossible to change "human nature" which is given and unalterable.

Weber saw that an ethic of responsibility was most difficult to

131. Weber, "Politics as a Vocation".
132. Ibid., p. 127.
133. Ibid., p. 124.
134. Ibid., p. 121.
135. Ibid., p. 128.

bear authentically. Indeed the qualities of the good politician include detachment, calmness, objectivity and distance from a reality which he perceives without benefit of illusion. Yet he must also be warm and passionate at the same time as being cool and proportionate.[136] These are very difficult to combine and the Sartrean "heroes", Hoederer and Goetz, are very much alone, detached and grim figures who are determined to pursue their chosen course of action. However, Hoederer accepts far more responsibility than does Goetz. *The Devil and the Good Lord* traces the development of Goetz from a narcissistic ethic of absolute ends to one of responsibility, of collective discipline on earth. He accepts responsibility because he can do no other! God is dead.

But how is an earthly salvation to be found? Sartre admires Hoederer most, and understands Hugo best since Hugo so resembles Sartre himself in many ways.[137] Hoederer is an existential man of action yet does not incarnate the reality of an autonomous individual. Goetz most certainly does not. The distinction between an ethic of responsibility and one of ultimate ends seems to be an important one in Sartre's political world. But those who accept an ethic of responsibility—Brunet, Goetz, Jean and Hoederer—are exactly those who seem part of a *corpus mysticum*. They do not have a personal reality - they are soldiers of a cause to which they are slaves and do not question it. The division seems to be between the communist intellectual of the P.C.F. and the bourgeois-anarchist intellectual who lives on the margin—he rejects his own class, but is not accepted by, nor does he belong to the other. The latter is lost and aimless, feeling unreal and discontinuous. His idealism for the Cause is narcissistic idealization. He acts as he does because of the intrinsic rightness of the act, yet also finds it difficult to act because he is not totally convinced on another level. Hugo cannot shoot Hoederer because, as Hoederer observes "an intellectual's always got to think",[138] and Hugo is frightened of soiling his hands. Hoederer tells Hugo:

> All right, stay pure! Who does it help and why did you come to us? Purity is an ideal for a fakir or a monk. You intellectuals, you bourgeois anarchists, you use it as an excuse for doing nothing.

These intellectuals, Hoederer tells Hugo, are not afraid of actions, of blood, but of "the rest"—the decision-making and the taking of

136. Ibid., pp. 115-16.
137. Contat and Rybalka, p. 183.
138. Sartre, *Crime Passionnel*, p. 104.

responsibility.[139] But Hoederer, Goetz and Brunet do not take the ultimate responsibility—responsibility for themselves. They incarnate only a relative ethic of responsibility—one which takes "effectiveness" as the criterion of action but does not question the nature of this "effectiveness". In comparison with the "bourgeois anarchists" whose ethic is one in which effectiveness does not figure, it is certainly much closer to an ethic of responsibility since effectiveness is the only criterion. Yet "effectiveness" is always effectiveness *for* something. This something is not a simple given objective end, but one chosen by people. The choice itself is free. The man who takes an ethic of responsibility seriously chooses not only effectiveness, but the end to which the means is efficacious.

The ethic of responsibility of Sartre's party men seems based on an ethic of ultimate ends. Sartre's criticism of the party has always been the way in which choice and freedom are curtailed in its organization. Once someone joins the Party, his mind and body belong to it;[140] he can only leave the Party feet first.[141] Organization and effectiveness on the one hand, and spontaneity and freedom on the other seem to be mutually exclusive in Sartre's political world. Neither way is authentic. This choice is conditioned as has been observed above, by the actual nature and position of the stalinist P.C.F. in particular, and the historical alternatives in general. It is not a pretty scene.

The world described seems to be one only of struggles for recognition. We are all nothingnesses, absences and even the range of political choices seem to be based on self-deception. Identity in the P.C.F. is symbiotic relation with the strong and powerful Party, the Cause, the idealized Proletariat. Out of the Party, the intellectual has nothing and is nothing—he is weak and impotent. The world is a closed system. A third autonomous party cannot enter or even get going, especially since autonomy can only be illusion. We are nothing and can define outselves only in relations of recognition—a recognition which is impossible since there is no personhood to recognize. There is no way out of our being appendages to the roles we play or assume. Hugo likes Slick, one of Hoederer's bodyguards, "because he's so strong and never thinks".[142] He tells Slick: "How

139. Ibid., p. 95.

140. "'When a man joins the Party, nothing but the Party matters', said Brunet." Sartre, *Iron in the Soul*, p. 340. "His words belonged to the Party; the Party alone gave to them any meaning they might have. Only within the party could Brunet love, persuade, console". Ibid., p. 346.

141. Sartre, *Crime Passionnel*, p. 81.

142. Ibid., p. 74.

lovely it must be inside your head; not a sound, a nice dark night".[143] Sartre obviously envies the simple soldier, the man who never questions anything, the child who plays with others in the park. They never think to question their existence, they are never aware of the deceptions on which their lives are based. The possibility of questioning one's position, of not deceiving oneself, at the same time leading a life which is worthwhile in its own right, does not enter Sartre's scheme of things on a personal level; and a political movement which does not devour its members, thus negating its professed ends, also seems impossible. Sartre's recent maoist, political activism seems an incarnation of Hugo rather than Hoederer, instead of a transcendence of the politics of both. Perhaps however, such a transcendence is not possible.

Since our existence is inevitably political—that is, conditioned by the workings of large social groupings—in Sartre's view we are always at the mercy of others. The only relations that seem to occur are those defined in terms of recognition, of torture, of conflict. They are sado-masochistic in systems seemingly run on hate. The only escape hatch is in solidarity with others against some mighty force. But then the individual becomes submerged in the group, losing any identity he may have formerly had. Sartre has always been fascinated with the rôle of the "third" to break the sado-masochistic game of recognition. But the "third" inevitably seem to go the way of the others. Nonetheless it seems to be for Sartre our only hope. Unhappily the third world acts as a screen for our projections and loses much of its purity in and after the battle. The third world seems to be defined in conflictual terms with the rest of the world—it does not have its own identity. Victory is seen as beating the persecutors, but what about identity if there were no enemies after victory? The alternatives Sartre sees are cast in terms of engulfment and defence against engulfment, thus constantly creating a negative identity. I have shown through examples how Sartre's view of politics seems conditioned by pre-oedipal problems of identity, how these concern primary processes together with external realities which they mirror at least in part. He confronts some of the problems of political action in an alienated world, and these can be seen on levels other than the purely political one.

In the next chapter I shall pursue the relations and possibilities of politics and psychology in the case of the development of a well-known figure whose work owes much to that of Sartre, and who also attempts to grapple with the realities and possibilities of our time: R.D. Laing.

143. Ibid., p. 76.

# PART II

# R.D. LAING

# 5

# The Mystification of an Imprisoned Soul

This chapter will attempt to show the comprehensibility of R.D. Laing's change in approach and views from his first book, *The Divided Self*, through to his mystical position, in terms of what seems to be Laing's essential project: namely, to make "insane" experience intelligible in terms of the agency both of the "patient" and of the context in which it is situated. Laing endeavours to show how the person designated "insane" is trying to make the best he can of an unlivable situation: insanity is a normal reaction to an insane context. This is not to say that the patient himself is sane, for he is often dreadfully affected by the situation. Nor is there an indication that biochemical elements never play a part.[1] Far more often than most psychiatrists imagine, Laing suggests, the "patient" is precipitated into "insanity" by his social milieu.

In *The Divided Self* Laing writes that the normal individual, when confronted with a situation which threatens his very being and which offers no escape

> develops a schizoid state in trying to get outside it, if not physically, at least mentally: he becomes a mental observer who looks on, detached and impassive, at what his body is doing or what is being done to his body. If this is so in the normal, it is at least possible to suppose that the individual whose abiding mode of being-in-the-world is of this split nature is living in what to him, if not to us, is a world that threatens his being from all sides, and from which there is no escape. This is indeed the case for such people. For them the world is a prison without bars, a concentration camp without barbed wire.[2]

1. Laing (1960); *The Divided Self: An Existential Study in Sanity and Madness*, (Preface to Pelican Edition, 1965), p.9. Laing's mystical position effectively ended on his return from Ceylon, and since then he has reverted to earlier positions for continuing his investigations. *See* Introduction.
2. Laing, *The Divided Self*, p.79.

This moving description of the schizoid state of being is central to Laing's writings. As the context of investigation broadens from the individual through to the total social world itself, the "normal" situation hitherto bracketed out of the inquiry becomes "schizoid". Finally the world itself is seen by Laing as it is seen by his schizoid of *The Divided Self.* The other, the family, the world come to be seen as threatening the individual's being. The only sane way to preserve individual experiencing—in an almost overwhelming situation—is a form of disembodiment, as the body is in the service of an oppressing and impinging reality.

The reality, formerly seen as potentially emancipatory, Laing now sees as inherently repressive. The schizophrenic of *The Politics of Experience*, who does not find living in the world as constituted for him a feasible proposition, may refuse it and embark on a voyage or journey unconfined by it. The Eastern mystic seeing the world as illusion may transcend it. To stay in the world is to remain imprisoned in it. Many "normals" are so far divorced from themselves that in their double alienation they do not realize just how imprisoned they are. The "mentally ill" are often in the odd position of not being able to function smoothly and "normally", and thus being in a position where certain questions about their existence actually come up and are able to be confronted. Laing himself, in his contribution to the Rochester International Conference on Schizophrenia in 1967, gave voice to the path described in this chapter.

> Everyone who has made a close study of the families of schizophrenics appears to agree that much, or even all, the apparent irrationality of the individual finds its rationality in the original family context. But the family as a whole appears irrational. However we may expect that the irrationality of the family will find *its* rationality when placed in *its* context. And so on ... presumably through meta-meta-meta- ... contexts, until one arrives at the contexts of all social contexts, the *Total World System* (TWS). This seems irrational enough, but may find its rationality in a further meta-context of which we have only vague intimations.[3]

It may be seen that there are a number of related dimensions through which Laing's explorations may be viewed. In this chapter the correlations of these dimensions will be noted as part of a unified project. Broadly the dimensions to be examined are intelligibility and breadth of context; characteristics of the context, including intellectual influences and changes in approach which Laing has brought

3. Laing (1967), "The Study of Family and Social Contexts in Relation to the Origin of Schizophrenia", p. 141.

to bear on them; the view of reality, embodiment and disembodiment, mental illness and schizophrenia, and sanity and insanity.

For present purposes this chapter divides Laing's work into five main stages characterized by their basic contexts. These foci are:

(i) *Self*-concentration on ontological security and insecurity, embodiment and disembodiment, true and false-self systems.[4]

(ii) *Self and Other*—interpersonal dynamics, stratagems.[5]

(iii) *The Family*—group dynamics, election of "mad" member.[6]

(iv) *The Total Social World System.*[7]

(v) *Transcendentalism*—contradiction, mysticism.[8]

4. Laing (1957), "An Examination of Tillich's Theory of Anxiety and Neurosis", *British Journal of Medical Psychology*, XXX, p. 88ff.
Laing, *The Divided Self.*
5. Laing (1961), *The Self and Others.*
R.D. Laing and A. Esterson (1958), "The Collusive Function of Pairing in Analytic Groups", *British Journal of Medical Psychology*, XXXI, pp. 117-23.
Laing (1954), "Practice and Theory—The Present Situation", Sixth International Congress of Psychotherapy. *Psychother-Psychosom* 13, pp. 58-67.
R.D. Laing, H. Phillipson, A.R. Lee (1966), *Interpersonal Perception: A Theory and Method of Research.*
Laing (1969), *Self and Others.*
6. Laing (1962), "Series and Nexus in the Family", *New Left Review* 45.
R.D. Laing and D.G. Cooper (1964), *Reason and Violence: A Decade in Sartre's Philosophy, 1950-1960.*
R.D. Laing and A. Esterson (1964), *Sanity, Madness and the Family: Families of Schizophrenics* (Preface to Second Edition, 1969).
Laing (1965), "Mystification, Confusion and Conflict", I. Boszormenyi—Nagy and J.L. Framo (eds.), *Intensive Family Therapy: Theoretical and Practical Aspects.*
Laing (1967), "Family and Individual Structure" in P. Lomas (ed.), *The Predicament of the Family.*
Laing (1967), "The Study of Family and Social Contexts in Relation to the Origin of Schizophrenia" in J. Romano (ed.), *The Origins of Schizophrenia.*
Laing (1969), *Self and Others.*
Laing (1971), *The Politics of the Family and Other Essays.*
7. Laing (1964), "One-Dimensional Man", *New Left Review.*
Laing (1964), "What is Schizophrenia?", paper read to the First International Congress of Social Psychiatry, *New Left Review.*
Laing (1967), "The Obvious" in D. Cooper (ed.) *The Dialectics of Liberation.*
Laing (1968), "Metanoia: Some Experiences at Kingsley Hall, London" in H.M. Ruitenbeek (ed.), *Going Crazy: The Radical Therapy of R.D. Laing and Others.*
Laing (1967), *The Politics of Experience and the Bird of Paradise. The Politics of Experience* falls within this category and the following—while *The Bird of Paradise* falls only within the following category.
8. Laing, *The Politics of Experience and the Bird of Paradise. See* 7.
Laing (1970), *Knots.*
Laing (1971), Quotes in interviews with P. Mezan, "After Freud and Jung, Now Comes R.D. Laing", *Esquire.* This article contains a great many statements by Laing in formal and informal encounters with Mezan during 1971. (Ctd next p.)

## (i) SELF

Laing wrote *The Divided Self* in 1955 when he was 28.[9] Its purpose was "to make madness and the process of going mad comprehensible".[10] This view of madness was in contrast with the prevailing view that there was a more or less firm distinction between the psychotic and the neurotic patient.[11] The neurotic's behaviour was able to be comprehended and changed while the psychotic's was regarded as totally bizarre, inappropriate, deluded, irresponsible and beyond all reason.

Laing's interest is not in all the psychoses, but in certain types of schizophrenic and schizoid behaviour. Schizophrenic states are the most commonly diagnosed mental illnesses in mental hospitals. Laing's own interest in "access to birth and death" decided his original interest in medicine;[12] his experiences in Glasgow Royal Mental Hospital[13] together with a great intellectual interest in existentialism,[14] particularly that of Sartre[15] and the work of certain British analysts followed.[16] It is worth noting that apart from self-evident organic disorders resulting in gross mental disturbance, schizophrenic psychoses constitute a paradigm for the application of the illness model in psychiatry. "It remains that central core of what we consider unreason or madness."[17] If this paradigm is upset, then much else goes too.

Laing (1973), Interview in *Rolling Stone*.

It will readily be seen that, on the face of it, the dates of some of his published works in the sections seem out of place *chronologically*. It should be noted that *The Politics of the Family* basically is a revised collection of essays published previously, and that *Self and Others* is a revision of *The Self and Others*, preserving the original focus. The characterization of Laing's work is one of his focal points of interest rather than chronological development, i.e. the foci are intellectual rather than necessarily chronological. Because Laing's work is taken as a project, it should not be surprising that there are often elements of other stages contained in each.

9. Laing, *The Divided Self*, p. 11.
10. Ibid., p. 9.
11. S. Freud, "The Unconscious" (1915) pt. 7 in P. Rieff (ed.), *Sigmund Freud: General Psychological Theory*.
12. Cited by Mezan, p. 156.
13. Ibid., pp. 168, 171.
14. Laing; *The Divided Self*, p. 10.
15. *See* frequent quotations from Sartre in *The Divided Self*, and in Charlesworth, *The Existentialists and Jean-Paul Sartre*, pp. 47-50.
16. Note, for example, Laing's use of the concept of "false self" and "false-self system" and Winnicott's "false self". The work of Fairbairn, a fellow-Scotsman whose work he was aware of, led him to a revaluation of psychotic illness. Winnicott, for example, had characterized schizophrenia in 1948 as "a sort of environmental deficiency". Winnicott, *Collected Papers*.
17. Romano, *The Origins of Schizophrenia*, p.1.

If the schizophrenic patient is viewed by the psychiatrist, from the start, as a person whose experience and behaviour he will try to understand sympathetically as being at least potentially contextually sensible behaviour aimed at achieving a reasonable adaptation, a different picture emerges. The patient is then not viewed purely as exhibiting psychopathology, which for practical purposes is treated as irrelevant to agency—like other medical diseases. Schizophrenic symptomatology may be used by some people to preserve a precariously structured self, the basic structure of which is established in early infancy.[18]

*The Divided Self* is a phenomenological investigation of schizoid experience—of what it is like to be schizoid or schizophrenic. Once the patient is regarded as a person and not simply as a resultant of certain mechanisms, the mode of his experience of himself and others can be investigated. Laing uses the term "ontological insecurity" to describe the continued base state of schizoid and schizophrenic experience. In contrast to the ontologically secure person, the ontologically insecure person experiences himself as "pre-occupied with preserving rather than gratifying himself: the ordinary circumstances of living threaten his *low threshold* of security". He feels dead, unreal, scarcely differentiated from the rest of the world "so that his identity and autonomy are always in question". He lacks temporal continuity, consistency, cohesiveness, substantiality and "he may feel himself as partially divorced from his body".[19]

The schizophrenic shut off from reality receives no supplies for his phantasy life from it.[20] Laing writes that the schizophrenic individual "is developing a microcosmos within himself; but of course, this autistic, private, intra-individual 'world' is not a feasible substitute for the only world there really is, the shared world. If this were a feasible project then there would be no need for psychosis".[21]

It may be seen that Laing does not envy the schizophrenic his position. Free only in phantasy and fettered in reality, the schizophrenic makes the best out of a disastrous situation, There is no doubt as to his insanity,[22] nor is there any doubt that he stands in need of psychotherapy to sort through his confusions and to try and achieve wholeness. Throughout *The Divided Self* Laing focusses on clinical material and on the way the classical psychoanalytic model does not

18. Laing, *The Divided Self*, p. 77.
19. Ibid., p. 42.
20. Ibid., p. 90.
21. Ibid., pp. 74-75.
22. Ibid., pp. 27,138.

properly fit the patients he describes. However, there is no crusade against psychoanalysis as such and the book abounds with psychoanalytic insights deriving from thc "English School". It is obvious that Laing regards enlightened psychotherapy as indicated at least for some schizoids and schizophrenics.

He emphasizes early infancy as a very important period for establishing later schizophrenia. Physical birth and existential birth do not necessarily coincide,[23] and for normal development, it is important that the mother and child recognize each other as distinct persons at a relatively early stage. "It is out of the earliest loving bonds with the mother that the infant develops the beginnings of a being-for-itself".[24] On the other hand the mothers of schizophrenics often do not allow this development[25] and the baby does not find the world feasible to be in. Not unreservedly but more than tentatively Laing suggests that although the first year of life with the mother is undoubtedly important, later relationships with father and siblings must not be forgotten with regard to schizophrenogenesis.[26] The emphasis on early thwarted relationship, especially with the mother, as being of great significance for the development of schizoidness and schizophrenia is very pronounced.

In *The Divided Self* neither the value nor the appropriateness of adaptation to "reality" is in question. Reality is the shared world of a common sense. It is what sane people take it to be, sanity being defined in terms of the reciprocal recognition of the other's identity and of the degree of conjunction or disjunction of two persons where the one is sane by common consent.[27] The real world of sane people, i.e. "the" world, is preferable to the private world of the schizoid. This is not to say that all those regarded as sane are less dangerous to themselves and others than those actually certified insane.[28] It does not mean that the presently constituted reality is a good one. But the emphasis of Laing in *The Divided Self* is not on problems connected with the "reality": this "reality" remains unquestioned, at least for the purposes of the investigation.

Related very much to the assumption of a common reality is the question of embodiment and disembodiment. To the extent that there is a disembodiment of the self, the person is schizoid. The sane person distinguishes his self/body from other. Whereas the schizoid

23. Ibid., p. 184.
24. Ibid., p. 190.
25. Ibid., p. 184.
26. Ibid., p. 190.
27. Ibid., pp. 35-36.
28. Ibid., p. 27.

person experiences a distinction between his self on one side and on the other his body and the rest of the world as bound together at a distance from him.[29] His body is not his in the same sense as another person is not him. Embodiment is one important feature of ontological security.[30] Reality is embodied reality.

Broader social issues are deliberately bracketed out of the inquiry of *The Divided Self.*

> It is the patient's life in her own interpersonal microcosmos that is the kernel of any psychiatric clinical biography. Such clinical biography is therefore self-consciously limited in scope. The socio-economic factors of the larger community of which the patient's family is an integral part are not *directly* relevant to the subject matter that is our concern. This is not to say that such factors do not profoundly influence the nature of the family and hence of the patient.[31]

Laing adds that no matter how different the social and class background of a particular patient who lives in the twentieth century western world

> very similar human possibilities arise in ... interpersonal relationships ... But we, as clinicians, must not forget that what goes on beyond our self-imposed horizons may make a great difference to the patterns to be made within the boundaries of our clinical interpersonal microcosms.[32]

The socio-economic-cultural background has been "temporarily placed in parenthesis for convenience" and the relevance in principle of these factors should not be forgotten.[33]

The stress is on the existential predicament of the individual and its resolution. Methodologically *The Divided Self* concentrates on the sanity or insanity of the individual person with secondary reference to significant others in his life. Laing quite simply is not commenting on socio-economic structure, but there is more than an indication that investigations which were methodologically focussed on a wider area could be revealing. The rest of the world is kept constant while the psychodynamics of the individual schizoid or schizophrenic are investigated. What is obvious though in *The Divided Self* is that there is an effect of the other or others on the schizoid and schizophrenic. The manner in which they affect him is not very clear. The inner experience of the schizoid or schizophrenic individual is primarily viewed in terms of internal rather than external dynamics.

29. Ibid., p. 82.
30. Ibid., p. 42.
31. Ibid., p. 180.
32. Ibid., pp. 180-81.
33. Ibid., p. 181.

### (ii) SELF AND OTHER

The focus of inquiry shifts from the intrapsychic problems of individual ontological security to interpersonal relationships. What self does to other and what other does to self assume importance. The subtitle of Laing's second book, *The Self and Others* (1961) is "Further studies in sanity and madness" indicating some continuity with *The Divided Self*. However the aim of this book is different:

> This book attempts to depict the own person within a social system or "nexus" of other persons; it attempts to understand the way in which the others affect his experience of himself and of them, and how accordingly his action takes shape.[34]

However Laing is not saying that "other people cause madness any more than a high hill can be the cause of heart failure in a sufferer from rheumatic heart disease".[35] As with *The Divided Self* in which Laing avowedly eschews any "comprehensive theory of schizophrenia",[36] Laing in *The Self and Others* offers no "aetiological theory of madness".[37] In *The Divided Self* Laing acknowledged his "main intellectual indebtedness" to the existential tradition[38] and this is revealed in his sympathetic rendering of individual schizoid expereince. In *The Self and Others* Laing gives a clue to a change of emphasis: although existentialist writers figure in the text and bibliography, Laing's main acknowledgements of sources are in two areas, that of psychoanalysis and psychoanalytically-oriented psychology, and that of American communications research.[39] The psychoanalysts referred to include Melanie Klein, Fairbairn and Winnicott, i.e. object-relations theorists whose views are by no means in contradiction with Laing's "existential" approach.[40]

The most important contribution of American communications theory to Laing was an article by Gregory Bateson, Don Jackson, Jay Haley and John Weakland entitled "Toward a Theory of

34. Laing, *The Self and Others*, p. ix.
35. Ibid., p. ix.
36. Laing, *The Divided Self*, p. 9.
37. Laing, *The Self and Others*, p. ix.
38. Laing, *The Divided Self*, p. 10.
39. Laing, *The Self and Others*, p. ix.
40. As Rycroft notes: "Existentialist philosophers and analysts criticize Freudian psychoanalysis on the ground that it neglects ontology and that its preoccupation with the past and with the unconscious has led it to neglect problems of consciousness and self-consciousness. These criticisms are characteristically levelled at instinct-theory and ego-psychology, and not at object-theory." C. Rycroft, *A Critical Dictionary of Psychoanalysis*, p. 107.

Schizophrenia"[41] in which the "double bind" thesis is first elaborated.[42] Bateson is an anthropologist at Palo Alto, Jackson is the Director and Haley edits *Family Process*. They are interested in a dynamic interactionist view of human relations. Communications research demonstrated the different levels, sometimes simultaneous but with opposing messages, that people convey to one another. This is illustrated well by Searles' paper, "The Effort to Drive the Other Person Crazy" (1959)[43] which is discussed by Laing.[44] The work of Erving Goffman should also be noted.[45]

According to Laing the most "significant theoretical and methodological developments in the psychiatry of the last two decades" has been in the field of inquiry into interactions of self and others, and the gradual displacing of "a basically monadic psychology"; one which treats the individual without reference to others, which "artificially isolates him from the context of his life, interpersonal and social".[46] "In Freud's theory ... one has the 'I' (ego) the 'over-me' (super-ego) and 'it' (id) but no *you*..." But "the world is peopled by others, and these others are not simply objects in the world: they are centres of reorientation in the objective universe. "Nor are these others simply other I's. The others are you, he, him, her, them, etc.[47] Psychiatry then has been guilty of a methodological individualism. Not only must the patient be treated as agent and his actions and words be taken seriously as valid (as with the schizophrenics in *The Divided Self*), but others must be taken seriously as others. Direction must be found not only from an orientation of person-centredness or subjectivity, but from the effects of other persons on the self. The other is another person. "In order to recognize persons and not simply objects, one must realize that the other human being is not only another object in space but another centre of orientation to the objective world."[48] A methodological shift of orientation is apparent in Laing from self to self and others.[49]

41. G. Bateson, et al, "Toward a Theory of Schizophrenia", *Behavioral Science*. I.
42. Laing, *The Self and Others*, p. 136 ff.
43. H. Searles, "The Effort to Drive the Other Person Crazy", *British Journal of Medical Psychology*. XXXII.
44. Laing, *The Self and Others*, Ch. 12.
45. E. Goffman, *Asylums: Essays on the Social Situation of Mental Patients and Other Inmates*.
46. Laing, *The Self and Others*, p. 69.
47. Laing et al, *Interpersonal Perception*, p. 3.
48. Laing, "Mystification, Confusion and Conflict", p. 347.
49. It is clear that Laing understood the difference in emphasis. Originally Laing intended to publish *The Divided Self* and *The Self and Others* as "two parts of a single book, but when I took it around to about five publishers, they all rejected it

As has been seen in Part I, Sartre had written voluminously about the relation of self and other, not only in *Being and Nothingness* but in his prose and theatre. "Hell is other people"—the other always poses a threat to my freedom. He defines me relegating me to object-status. Relationships are sado-masochistic.[50] All human relationships are locked in tension and conflict. Life is a constant struggle to absorb others and resist being absorbed by them. In *Huis Clos*, the dead, who are now defined forever as solely what they have been, are given the chance to leave their conflict-ridden and intrinsically frustrating prison when the door opens. But nobody leaves. In fact one of the prisoners closes the door.[51] For Sartre as for Laing the world is a prison without bars. Most dramatic is the second-empire drawing room of *Huis Clos* (originally entitled *Les Autres*) which has no window, no glass and an electric light that cannot be extinguished. Everybody is condemned to wait for ever. In *Altona* Franz only leaves his room to suicide with his father. Immediately his place is taken by his sister, the equilibrium is restored. In nearly all of Sartre's plays, Boros observes, one is struck by one characteristic of the decor: the action always takes place in a closed room.[52] In *Being and Nothingness* the other takes my freedom, imprisoning me by his gaze, and in the *Critique* one is also under the domination of the group, not only because defined in their eyes but as always one too many. For Sartre, life is itself a prison.[53] Despite Sartre's explicit denial,[54] Mauriac's statement that it is Sartre himself who is the *séquestré* may contain much truth.[55] Can the same be said of Laing?

The motto of *The Self and Others* is a quotation from Confucius which asks this same question: "The way out is via the door. Why is it that no one will use this method?". Laing answers basically that it is impossible to leave because the individual is trapped in a phantasy system involving others who would strongly disapprove and might even label one "bad" or "mad" for attempting to leave.[56] According to Laing most people hold tenable positions within phantasy systems

because it was too big and suggested that I redo it as two books". (Laing in Mezan, p. 171). The contexts of investigation are different in the two books, yet connected by a single project.

50. Sartre, *Being and Nothingness*, Part Three, Ch. 3.
51. *See* Ch. 2 of the present work.
52. Boros, *Un séquestré: l'homme sartrien*, p. 2.
53. S. Doubrovsky, "Sartre and Camus: A Study in Incarceration", p. 92.
54. Sartre, Interview with O. Pucciani.
55. Cited in Boros, p. 10.
56. Laing, *Self and Others*, pp. 42-43.

of a nexus. "This is normally called having an 'identity' or 'personality'. We never realize we are in it. We never even dream of extricating ourselves. We tolerate, punish, or treat as harmless, bad or mad those who try to extricate themselves and tell us we should also."[57] These individuals occupy what Laing calls "an untenable position" since they can neither stay nor leave. And the more they occupy this position the further they are from getting out of it. "As one person's experience of a situation he is in with others comes to be more disjunctive with those of the others in the "sane" situation, his actions become more and more dissonant with actions of the others."[58] As the positions become more entrenched they spiral into what Laing describes as "the most extreme interexperiential disjunction in our culture—psychiatrists sane: patients psychotic".[59] Interexperiential events are regarded as intra-psychic pathology. Psychoanalysis does not recognize that the individual interacts with others and only takes the individual's action into account, discounting others' reactions or initiating actions.[60] Out of context the individual's actions can be seen as mad. Another way of putting this is to say that individual's are involved in games with others, and breaking the rules of the game or playing a different one can be regarded as neurotic or psychotic. Laing points to the contributions of the American psychiatrists Eric Berne and Thomas Szasz in illuminating this approach.[61] Transactional analysis focusses on interpersonal game-playing, on the effects self and other have on each other.

With the introduction of the other into the context it becomes possible to introduce different explanations for certain forms of behaviour of self often considered pathological. When the other is introduced, it becomes clear that pathological behaviour is pathological behaviour as seen by somebody else, which points to the fact that perception involves a selection of data which are part of the phantasy system of the person ascribing pathology.[62] In fact, self and other may subscribe to the same or different phantasy systems. But in any case a microcosmos or what is termed "reality" is set up. What is real to one person may not be to another, or it may be real to both of them and unreal to everyone else or vice versa. What someone considers private another sees publicly. What someone sees

57. Ibid., p. 41.
58. Ibid., p. 42.
59. Ibid., p. 43.
60. Laing et al, *Interpersonal Perception*, p. 8.
61. Ibid., pp. 7-8.
62. Ibid., p. 10.

as outside him, another sees as "in" him. "The World" is not exactly the same for any two people.[63] There is no clinically detached, objective observer of clinical objective facts. One person investigating the experience of another can be directly aware only of his own experience of the other. Laing puts the reasonably firm reality of *The Divided Self* up for question. What one regards as real or unreal is to a large extent a function of what group one is in. And "all groups operate by means of phantasy".[64]

Given a distinction between experience and behaviour, within the group itself others will experience self's behaviour in a different way from the way that self does. And self's identity "undergoes myriad metamorphoses or alterations, in terms of the others I become to the others".[65]

"We can see that in a dyadic system there is no isolated individual person. The one person, in order to maintain *his own* self-identity, has to *act towards the other* and however adroit a strategist he may be, he can never rely on controlling the other."[66] The inherent impingement of other on self is evident: self and other are in constant irresolvable conflict. Self preserves his identity *against* other. Self and other may find themselves in ascending "manic" spirals, or in descending "depressive" ones in which one or both are attempting to escape from false or untenable positions.[67]

Is it possible for self and other to have a genuine meeting? Laing, like Sartre, answers in the negative. Even where both partners want such a meeting, mutual trust, confidence, vulnerability and confirmation are required. "Desire for confirmation from each is present in both, but each is caught between trust and mistrust, confidence and despair and both settle for counterfeit acts of confirmation on the basis of pretence. To do so *both* must play the game of collusion."[68] Collusion is a game in which it is vital that the partners do not admit that it is a game. In *Les Mains sales* Sartre faces the problem:

> **Hugo**: Jessica, try to understand. Be serious.
> **Jessica**: Why should I be serious?
> **Hugo**: Because we can't play all the time.
> **Jessica**: I don't like being serious, but I'll try.
> I'll play at being serious.

63. Laing, *Self and Others*, p. 36.
64. Ibid., p. 39.
65. Laing et al, *Interpersonal Perception*, p. 4.
66. Ibid., p. 27. (Cf. Sartre.)
67. Ibid., p. 32.
68. Laing, *Self and Others*, pp. 108-9.

This scene devoted to the possibility of collusion ends:

> **Hugo**: You're playing at being serious. You said so.
> **Jessica**: No, you said so.
> **Hugo**: You must believe me—please you must believe me.
> **Jessica**: I'll believe you if you'll believe I'm serious.
> **Hugo**: All right, I'll believe you.
> **Jessica**: No, you're only playing at believing me.[69]

"The one person does not use the other merely as a hook to hang projections on. He strives to find in the other, or to reduce the other to become, the very *embodiment* of projection." Collusion is

> always clinched when self finds in other that other who will "confirm" self in the false self that is trying to make real and vice versa. The ground is then set for prolonged mutual evasion of truth and true fulfilment. Each has found an other to endorse his own false notion of himself and to give this appearance a semblance of reality.[70]

Collusion, on the face of it, seems to be as close to a genuine encounter as is possible, since other threatens self's integrity by his very existence, and vice versa. Both bolster each other in their self-deceptions. But the problem is that a third may threaten the collusion.[71] As Sartre says in *Being and Nothingness*, the pair may be fixed by the look of a third. The subjectivity of each is transformed into object-status for the third. The "bad faith" of the collusive partners is revealed. Laing refers to *Huis Clos* which he says "reveals the agony of failure to sustain identity when the project of one's life is such that a tolerable self-identity requires collusion.[72] He also discusses Genet's play, *The Balcony*[73] implicitly agreeing with Genet's conclusion that collusive make-believe is the stuff of our lives. Examples of collusion in analytic group situations are attested.[74] It is not possible, according to Laing, to abolish collusion since all groups embody phantasy systems. The point is rather to change the perspective such that, and he refers to a Zen master, the attempt to abolish collusion *per se* is given up. "Therapy without collusion cannot help but frustrate desires generated by phantasy."[75]

Laing's view of the intrinsic hostility of other is further elucidated

69. Sartre, *Crime Passionnel*, p. 34.
70. Laing, *Self and Others*, p. 111.
71. Ibid., p. 111.
72. Ibid., p. 112.
73. Ibid., pp. 112-18.
74. Ibid., pp. 118-24. Laing and Esterson; "The Collusive Function of Pairing in Analytic Groups".
75. Laing, *Self and Others*, p. 124.

in his taking over of the double-bind theory of Bateson *et al* and his articulation of Searles' paper "The Effort to Drive the Other Person Crazy". The violence other perpetrates on self, even if unknown to either, is enormous. It is most apparent with the schizophrenic "victim" of a situation in which he is required to do or think contradictory things neither of which is right. Withdrawal from the situation is also wrong. Failure is assured, but a schizoid withdrawal may be the most adaptive stratagem for the "victim" of contradictory demands, attributions, etc. Laing regards the work of the Palo Alto group as having "revolutionized" the meaning of "environment", especially with regard to the origins of schizophrenia.[76] The environment of the incipient schizoid or schizophrenic person is the common phantasy world of the others of his family in relation to him. It is impossible for the incipient schizoid to obey the instructions which would allow him to accord with the prevalent phantasy system. However it is sometimes possible for this individual to play at or pretend to act in accord with this system, assuming different guises at different times. This person will present one or many faces to "the world", his true self locked as far away as possible from the danger others present. What else can he do in a situation where he is free to leave, but God help him if he does, and if he stays he is in as much trouble? Similarly, Searles explains how a person may be driven crazy by contradictory communications tending "to undermine the other person's confidence in his own emotional reactions and his own perceptions of reality".[77] Laing sees these modes as "mystifying" as he does the "double bind" situation.[78]

Within the nature of reality as a function of phantasy systems, Laing's concern with embodiment as a central feature of sanity diminishes. The body is not simply body, but body-for-someone. Since the dichotomies of inner and outer; mental and physical; mental activities and external and bodily realities; figments and what can be touched, handled, seen; psychical reality and physical reality; inner mind and external bodily development, and finally the division of mind and body[79] are all up for phenomenological questioning, Laing's concern with self as a bodily self in *The Divided Self* disappears. The false-self system of *The Divided Self* is now constituted by the expectations of the other, to which self conforms. One starts from the individual's experience without theoretical presuppositions

76. Ibid., p. 148.
77. Cited in Laing, *Self and Others*, p. 139.
78. Laing, "Mystification, Confusion and Conflict", pp. 352-53.
79. Laing, *Self and Others*, pp. 23-24.

as to the constitution of the individual who is experiencing.[80] Phenomenologically my body appears for me in "dreams, imagination and memory" as "alive or dead, real or unreal, whole or in bits".[81] My body-for-self may not be private in another's phantasy. I may lose an area of unqualified privacy which is often "associated with the process of going mad" and Laing goes on to assure the reader that this is not connected with "loss of ego-boundary" or disembodiment as in *The Divided Self* but with his view of "reality" or "the world".[82] Embodiment has lost priority to what the poet Gerald Manley Hopkins describes as "my self-being, my consciousness and feeling of myself, that taste of myself, of *I* and *me* above and in all things" which is very distinctive and incommunicable to others.[83]

In *The Divided Self* sane and schizoid positions are defined in terms of whether self is embodied or not. In Laing's focus on self and other, the body receives hardly a mention and where it is referred to it is in the context of challenging self's relation to body as particularly important.

In the focus on self and other, the notion of sanity itself receives scant attention. No definition of what it is is offered: only a statement of what it is not.. A patient was told by his father that whether he was his son depended on whether his father regarded him as such at the particular time. The patient internalized this to mean that he, the patient, was who he said he was and not who he said he was not. Laing remarks: "True sanity lies at the other side: the negation of the psychotic negation of the false original premise. I am not what they say I am, nor what I say I am."[84] In *Interpersonal Perception* Laing is concerned not with sane or insane positions, but with the level of mutual understanding of self and other. Interestingly too, the subtitle of *The Self and Others*, "Further Studies in Sanity and Madness" was dropped from the second edition—*Self and Others* (1969). In a world where self is imprisoned with hostile others, how is sanity possible? It seems more that

> one should know the social risks if one makes a break with social reality: if one begins deliberately to make a systematic attempt not to be the self that everyone takes one to be to escape from this identity by playing at that everyone takes one to be, to escape from this identity by playing at not being there, by being anonymous, or incognito, adopting pseudonyms, saying one is dead, saying one is nobody because one's body does not belong to oneself.[85]

80. Ibid., pp. 25-27.
81. Ibid., pp. 34-35.
82. Ibid., p. 36.
83. Hopkins quoted in ibid., p. 35.
84. Laing, *Self and Others*, pp. 96-97.
85. Ibid., p. 53.

## (iii) THE FAMILY

Laing and Cooper characterize the work of Sartre they are concerned with in *Reason and Violence* as just "as important for demystification of the present as Freud's and Marx's formulations, for instance, were in their day".[86] The *Critique de la raison dialectique* and *Question de methode* (*Search for a Method*) were published together in 1960, and *Saint Genet* was published as far back as 1952. Laing wrote a short article on the *Critique* in 1962,[87] in which he acknowledges the theory of the *Critique* as having been "of immense help to me in my own researches, both practically and specifically into families, and more theoretically and generally".[88] In 1964, Laing and Aaron Esterson published some of this type of research in *Sanity, Madness and the Family* and in the same year Laing and David Cooper published *Reason and Violence*.[89] Laing and Cooper present *Saint Genet* as "perhaps the most radical attempt by one man to understand the life of another living man in its most basic forms recorded in literature".[90] Though transitional, *Saint Genet* is to be understood in the theoretical context of the *Search for a Method* and the *Critique*.[91] "All Genet's relations with the other, as Sartre describes them, are *group relations*."[92]

The *Critique* focusses on the primacy of the group in human living. The early Sartre centred on self and relations with others. The *Critique* depasses *Being and Nothingness*: "The key positions of the earlier work are conserved ... through a dialectical transformation as one moment in the later synthesis".[93]

A group begins to be formed when a number of people are bracketed together as one social entity, not a number of individuals.[94] To write now of an unmediated self relating to other is an abstraction, for self and other are already themselves grouped and

86. Laing and Cooper, *Reason and Violence*, p. 10.
87. Laing, "Series and Nexus in the Family".
88. Ibid., p. 7.
89. In an unusual gesture Sartre himself has explicitly approved *Reason and Violence* in a Foreword to the work. Sartre wrote that he had the great pleasure in finding in it a very clear exposition of his work which remained true to his thought. Sartre even commends the authors' perfect understanding of the *Critique* and further praises the research of Laing and Cooper which he says contributes to the time "when psychiatry will be at last human". (my trans.) Sartre, Foreword to Laing and Cooper; *Reason and Violence*, p. 7.
90. Laing and Cooper, *Reason and Violence*, p. 27.
91. Ibid., p. 27.
92. Ibid., p. 17.
93. Ibid., p. 17.
94. Ibid., p. 12.

mediated through group experiences and structures.[95] What goes on in the group is always intelligible in terms of praxis, even the praxis of individuals. But these individuals are themselves in situation and have a group past. Sometimes what the group does appears as process, as though nobody is doing it. But this alienated praxis is to be traced back to the doers perhaps outside that group if it is to be intelligible, from "what is going on" (process) to "who is doing what" (praxis).[96] Such is the case when "free-floating actions, vagabonds without authors" are produced.[97] The group can act only through its members[98] and "is nothing but a multiplicity of relations and relations between relations".[99] Man in general is able to depass a situation, to be able "to do or undo what is done to him".[100] Praxis is "the passage from the objective through interiorization to the objective".[101] Even personal life is "a synthetic unity of what we make of what we are made of".[102] Every individual is born into a group which has already made pledges or commitments for him.[103] His conduct is limited and conditioned by the group rules. It is of course a mistake to view individual action as if it were not taking place in a group situation which has its own rules.[104]

The pledged group corresponds to what Laing refers to as a "nexus",[105] which he defines as "a group whose unification is achieved through the reciprocal interiorization by each of each other, in which neither a 'common object', nor organizational or institutional structures, etc. have a primary function as a kind of group 'cement' ... The unity of the nexus is the unification made by each person of the plurality of syntheses".[106] It exists "only in so far as each person incarnates the nexus. The nexus is everywhere, in each person, and is nowhere else than in each."[107] The family, in so far as it is nexal thus depends on the internalizations of each member of its structures.

95. Ibid., pp. 16, 151, 167.
96. Laing, "Series and Nexus in the Family", pp. 7-8.
105. Laing, "Series and Nexus in the Family", p. 11.
98. Ibid., p. 147.
99. Ibid., p. 48.
100. Ibid., p. 57.
101. Ibid., p. 53.
102. Ibid., p. 23.
103. Ibid., p. 144.
104. Ibid., p. 149.
105. Laing, "Series and Nexus in the Family", p. 11.
106. Ibid., p. 11.
107. Ibid., p. 12.

> If there is no external danger (to provide its *raison d'être*), then danger and terror have to be invented and maintained. Each member has to act on the others to maintain the nexus *in them* ... The stability of the nexus is the product of terror generated in its members by the work (violence) done by the members of the group on each other. Such family "homeostasis" is the product of reciprocities mediated under the statutes of violence and terror.[108]

According to Laing the nexal family's highest ethic is reciprocal concern of each member for each other's actions. The family then operates as a protection racket in which each is offered "protection-security against the violence that each threatens the other with, if anyone steps out of line".[109] Each person's need is not to have that need satisfied, but to have the others needing him to satisfy their needs. This is impossible, and spirals are set up. Nobody can be satisfied or fulfilled—a most unhappy situation.[110]

The opposite polarity of the nexus is the series. In a series, each is united with the other through a common relation to an object, and at the same time, through not being involved with each other in any other way, a negative unity. The serial group is a plurality of solitudes, of reciprocal indifference. Each is serial other to the others, and "repudiates his identity as a member of the group" in an alienated praxis. In a serial family situation each acts in terms of what "everyone" else would think or do. "There is conformity to a presence that is everywhere elsewhere".[111] Concrete family groups are, to a greater or lesser extent, a combination of nexus and series but normally principally nexal. According to Laing, then, family members can never be accepted for what they are. Each is under the reign of the violence and hostility of the others, denying him a personal identity.

*Sanity, Madness and the Family* is an attempt to provide a dialectical intelligibility for what happens in certain families, a (female) member of which had been hospitalized as schizophrenic. The intelligibility required is a translucency, a demystification, even a "diagnosis" or "seeing through" the family situation in terms of group dynamics and of the lived experience of the actors. This meant among other things that not only the family as a group was to be understood but also employing the concept of nexus in particular to what the family was for each of its members, what

108. Ibid., pp. 112-13.
109. Ibid., p. 13.
110. Ibid., pp. 13-14.
111. Ibid., pp. 9-11.

the family and its members were for members in certain combinations, as well as what the relations of these members were with each other. The world of the family was explored. What was hitherto considered to be the pathological process of one member designated schizophrenic was to be illuminated through a tracing back of this to the praxis of the family group itself. That is, the "pathology" of schizophrenia was found to be intelligible in terms of the social phenomenology of the family "world". Individual "madness" is dissolved in the broader context.

It should be made clear what Laing and Esterson claim to be doing here. In the Preface to the Second Edition, they point out that a control group of "normal" families is strictly irrelevant to *their* question which is: "Are the experience and behaviour that psychiatrists take as symptoms and signs of schizophrenia more socially intelligible than has come to be supposed?"[112] This is not to deny the interest that such a control group might have, but even if this projected group revealed the same sorts of interactions (which is unlikely given the fact that the status of schizophrenia is not that of a biochemical fact or strictly medical disease), this would not show the situation in families of schizophrenics to be less understandable *socially*. For example, certain social situations might predispose particular biochemical or genetic propensities toward schizophrenia to become filled, whereas in a similar situation where these predispositions were not present, this would not be so. The study of families of schizophrenics highlights the social interactions and alterations of family members. Strategies regarded as legitimate, and even necessary, within the family's "world" might be regarded as illegitimate and even crazy by others, outside that group. As Sartre had pointed out, irrationality is irrationality "for us" and not "in itself".[113]

Laing and Esterson in fact claimed to have discovered that schizophrenic symptoms could be intelligible in terms of social praxis.[114] They regard the shift of emphasis from individual pathology to their standpoint as of "historical significance no less radical than the shift from a demonological to a clinical standpoint three hundred years ago".[115] This is in line with Laing and Cooper's estimation of the work of the later Sartre, whose major concepts Laing and Esterson employ.[116] Also the American communications theorists

112. Laing and Esterson, *Sanity, Madness and the Family*, p. 12.
113. Laing and Cooper, *Reason and Violence*, p. 58.
114. Laing and Esterson, *Sanity, Madness and the Family*, pp. 34, 103.
115. Ibid., p. 27.
116. Ibid., p. 22.

who had previously influenced Laing, as well as the American researchers into families of schizophrenics, are acknowledged as of considerable help in their study.[117] Their view that schizophrenia is not a medical, pathological fact is in line with much current psychiatric research. For example, an Editorial Brief in *The Australian and New Zealand Journal of Psychiatry* states;

> It is probable that in the present state of our ignorance we are not justified in regarding schizophrenia as an illness or a disease, since the use of these words suggests that we have knowledge about its fundamental nature which we are in fact lacking.[118]

But it should be noted that the schizophrenics of *Sanity, Madness and the Family* are markedly different from those of *The Divided Self.* They do not speak "schizophrenese", and are very coherent. They are the "victims" of a group terror, rather than lacking inner ontological security (which was related with what happened in the first year of life). The schizophrenic of *Sanity, Madness and the Family* appears not to have very much to do with causing or creating some of the mystifications. The designated schizophrenic appears as passive recipient of the terror of the others to whom he can only react. In *The Divided Self*, the onset of schizophrenic symptoms would *ipso facto* change the family situation and create other reactions. The schizophrenic of *Sanity, Madness and the Family* seems nothing more than the scapegoat for the rest of the group. The schizophrenic does not seem in need of psychoanalytical treatment or relationship therapy as in *The Divided Self* at any rate no more than the rest of his family. As Laing had observed in *The Divided Self*, the "delusions" of the schizophrenic could be "literally true within the terms of reference of the individual who makes them".[119] The context and methodology have broadened considerably in *Sanity, Madness and the Family*, and much "delusion" falls into place as intelligible in terms of the violence done on the patient by the family group.

The family scene is seen by Laing not as an object but as a *drama*. Each member is an actor on the stage as well as a critic in the audience.[120] The drama has been carried out over many generations and carries across generations.[121]

117. Ibid., pp. 9-10.
118. *Australian and New Zealand Journal of Psychiatry* IV, p. 119.
119. Laing, *The Divided Self*, p. 149.
120. Laing, "Family and Individual Structure", p. 123.
121. Ibid., p. 110. Laing, *The Politics of the Family*, p. 86.

The critics in the audience, however, have not bought tickets: they are part of the cast itself. The participants in the situation cannot be assumed to know what is going on: the situation must be dis-closed. In fact, no one knows what the situation is.[122]

The family is characterized by an internalized system of reciprocal coinherences. It is a common "we" against the other "them".[123] "To be in the same family means having the same 'family' inside oneself."[124] The internalized patterns of relationship are incarnations of the family group structure.[125] In the family structure "each person in turn is ... a synthesiser of the interaction of the others, and finds himself synthesised into a social object in the course of similar interactions by another or others. Each person as a third party has a relation to each other as third, different in kind from the relation that each has with each as interactor being synthesised into a dyad *by* a third".[126] Laing writes elsewhere, "We cannot expect to catch the curtain going up or down in a drama we are born into. But there are plays within plays."[127] There are syntheses each makes of the others serially, but each is part of the situation being synthesised. Even the "plays within plays" are seen by a player in the role of a critic. The whole drams itself is beyond the observation of the players themselves. No wonder that Laing questions the "inner/outer" distinctions as misleading[128] in a web of reciprocal attributions, perceptions, internalizations and projections among a large number of members—especially where the family is smoothly running. These families may be the most mystified. These may be a "transpersonal system of collusion".[129]

The scenarios for the drama are set by the family's microhistory—the "terrain" between individual biography and large-scale history.[130] By processes of mapping past on to present and future, of structures of relationships being mapped on to other ones (nexification inducing others into our games and vice versa), and through operations of mystification, the family's microsocial world system becomes the fundamental reality for its members through the prism of which all else is viewed and acted on.

The mystified person operates in terms already mystified for

122. Laing, *The Politics of the Family*, pp. 31-35.
123. Ibid., p. 41. D. Cooper (ed.) *The Dialectics of Liberation*, p. 12.
124. Laing, "Family and Individual Structure", p. 119.
125. Laing, *The Politics of the Family*, p. 8.
126. Laing, "Family and Individual Structure", pp. 108-9.
127. Laing, *The Politics of the Family*, p. 86.
128. Laing, "Family and Individual Structure", p. 113.
129. Laing, *The Politics of the Family*, p. 99.
130. Ibid., p. 49.

him,[131] just as the actor finds his place within the terms of the scenario. Reality is the group reality. The drama is the frame of reference but in terms of the mystifications, the actor does not recognize his self-identity as *actor* in a drama. The group mystification is a form of praxis, albeit alienated, not a pathological process.[132] The actor does not know he is acting in the group praxis of the drama.

In *The Politics of the Family* in particular, Laing attempts to unravel the terms of the group phantasy system drama. He tries to uncover the mystifying operations involved in the attempts to keep a relative homeostasis of the family nexus, to ensure that "reality" remains intact. The scenarios and dramas are denied existence. First there are rules, then meta-rules which deny the existence of these rules and finally meta-meta-rules which deny their own existence as well as of those of the meta-rules and the rules. Such "govern the whole social field" and unless we can "see *through* these rules, we can only *see* through them".[133] According to Laing: "Rules govern all aspects of experience, *what* we are to experience, and what *not* to experience, the operation we must and must not carry out, in order to arrive at a permitted picture of ourselves and others in the world".[134] Yet meta-meta-rules and meta-rules prevent our seeing this as so.

> We are acting parts in a play that we have never read and never seen, whose plot we don't know, whose existence we can glimpse but whose beginning and end are beyond our present imagination and conception.[135]

The more "normal" or involved in the drama of life we become, the more alienated and mystified we are, the more adjusted within the family context, the tighter the knot. The less we see the inherent violence and terror in the nexus, the more "real" and "sane" we become. The most "normal" are the most mystified, and conversely.

In this situation, according to Laing, psychiatry plays a repressive role. Those who "see through" the mystifications are "outlawed and excommunicated" and "undergo secondary transformations".[136] Paraphrasing Laing, the psychiatrists (mind-police) diagnose an illness (crime) whereupon the patient (criminal) is hospitalized (imprisoned) and investigations follow. The patient (criminal) is convicted and sentence is passed (therapy). Those with a poor prognosis are dealt with as such, but most at the end of treatment (release) are

131. Laing, "Mystification, Confusion and Conflict", p. 353.
132. Ibid., p. 350.
133. Laing, *The Politics of the Family*, p. 105.
134. Ibid., p. 107.
135. Ibid., p. 87.
136. Ibid., p. 74.

adjusted (or obey the law) in future.[137] Obviously, Laing basically characterizes psychiatry as a violent criminal activity upon the self, forcing him to conform. It is not seen even potentially as healing, as bringing the person to wholeness as it is in *The Divided Self.*

It should scarcely be surprising then that Laing's attitude to the schizophrenic himself is different in this phase. Schizophrenia is a derogatory ascription by psychiatrists of a condition which they claim is pathological. But assuming pathology is self-validating, perhaps "much research into the origins of schizophrenia is hunting a hare whose origins may be in the mind of the hunters".[138] Laing believes the institutionalization of the "pathology" causes much of "schizophrenic" behaviour and refers to the work of Scheff, Goffman, Foucault and Szasz in this area.[139] Taken out of the family context the "schizophrenic's" behaviour is a cause of "schizophrenia". But to what extent does "schizophrenia" cause his subsequent hehaviour? Laing surmises that "normals" treated as "schizophrenics" would develop "schizophrenic" symptoms, and vice versa.[140] He quotes his own work at Kingsley Hall and David Cooper's Villa 21 as illustrating how people treated as "schizophrenic" can become well.[141] But such are normally prevented from doing so by "treatment" like ECT or psychotropic drugs. Laing suggests that the "schizophrenic" go through a "metanoia" (change of mind)[142] which resembles a voyage toward a rebirth and reintegration. What is often regarded as the beginnings of schizophrenic illness to be treated by cold packs, ECT and so on is in fact the "possible beginning of becoming well".[143] Healing is prevented instead of encouraged. The schizophrenic, who often regresses, is not tolerated by the society.[144]

Schizophrenia itself, writes Laing, is

> a kind of conceptual straitjacket, that severely restricts the possibilities both of psychiatrists and patients. Observations of animal behaviour in captivity indicate nothing reliable about their natural behaviour. The

137. Ibid., p. 74.
138. Laing, "The Study of Family and Social Contexts in Relation to the Origin of Schizophrenia", p. 139.
139. Laing, "Metanoia". Gordon, "Who is Mad? Who is Sane?".
140. Laing, "The Study of Family and Social Contexts in Relation to the Origin of Schizophrenia", pp. 140-41. Laing, *The Politics of the Family*, pp. 46-47.
141. Laing, *The Politics of the Family*, pp. 47-58. Laing, "The Study of Family and Social Contexts...", pp. 141-43.
142. Laing, "The Study of Family and Social Contexts...", p. 142.
143. Laing, *The Politics of the Family*, p. 52.
144. Ibid., p. 56.

observations psychiatrists base their view of schizophrenia on have, almost entirely, been made on human beings in a double or even treble capativity.[145]

The celebrated Mary Barnes, who had been through the gamut of ordinary psychiatric treatment, was regarded as an incurable schizophrenic. Finally, she became a resident of Kingsley Hall, and with the aid of Laing, his colleagues and other residents, went through a regression and emerged with some improvement.[146]

Schizophrenia in this stage has little to do with embodiment. The body receives scarcely a mention in this phase of Laing's development. At best it is the "range for introjective mappings from all domains".[147] Mental disturbances seem to have little to do with disembodiment. Here the body is merely a vehicle for the self.

Schizophrenics have been caught in a web, or a knot. They are trying to get out. Most people regard the process of realizing what is happening in their family nexus as threatening. They punish those like the schizophrenics who begin to "see through" the group nexus. Most people live in a hypnotic trance and those who try to wake from this state are punished as sick because they break the rules by seeing them. Psychiatrists even treat them for waking up, and drug them to sleep or "normality" again.[148] When the drama is seen as a drama by the "schizophrenic" who is only as much a player as the others—and no more—this threatens the rest of the players who do not wish to see themselves as playing. If they are just playing, what is left? So the schizophrenic is punished for not playing at being a player who does not know he is playing.[149]

145. Laing, "The Study of Family and Social Contexts in Relation to the Origin of Schizophrenia", p. 56.
146. Her account of what happened, together with that of her therapist, Joseph Berke, may be found in M. Barnes and J. Berke, *Mary Barnes: Two Accounts of a Journey Through Madness*.
147. Laing, *The Politics of the Family*, p. 117.
148. Ibid., p. 81.
149. Interestingly, Laing writes on situations and theory but not on therapy. Laing's actual therapeutic technique is reasonably orthodox. In Kingsley Hall "those few individuals who were in psychotherapy with Laing or one of the other therapists had their sessions elsewhere", writes Joseph Berke in Barnes and Berke, p. 233. Writes Mezan: "... for all the accusing rumours that (Laing) colludes in his patients' fantasies, or that he brings too much of the outside world into the consulting room, or that he is too motherly, or not motherly enough, patients of his assure me that, at least as an analyst, Laing's technique is scarcely less tough or orthodox than those of other virtuoso Freudians of a lesser notoriety". Mezan, p. 97. Also see Laing's comments in Charlesworth, *The Existentialists and Jean-Paul Sartre*.
Freud, according to Laing, is "the best of psychiatric writers" (*see* Gordon).

For Sartre, man's situation is defined by need and scarcity:

> Under the empire of scarcity human beings are seen as excess, as future consumers, as unnecessary at least, as a threat more fundamentally. Men are seen as quantities, as interchangeable. Man is put in question in his being; each is one-too-many. Each man exists as an inhuman, as a strange species, as other than me. The other is a risk for me. I am a risk for the other.[150]

In this situation,

> the scandal is ... in each person's perception of the other as one-too-many through interiorized scarcity. Under the rubric of interiorized scarcity the rationality of the *praxis* of each is the rationality of violence. Here violence is not a simple, naive ferocity of man, but the comprehensible reinteriorization of each of the contingent fact of scarcity.[151]

Sartre thus sees hostility and violence as constitutive of the human situation. There is a hint at the end of *Critique* of the possibility of a situation where this is not so; perhaps what Sartre terms a "third" can intervene in the struggle. Yet where is this "third" to come from? Nothing in the *Critique*, nor indeed anything else written by Sartre can make this "third" an intelligible possibility.

In *Huis Clos* the characters are eternally imprisoned in a stifling room the door out of which is locked. When it opens, Garcin finds it necessary to close it again: each is imprisoned by the others. In the *Critique* locked rooms are dispensed with. Even in the broad daylight, man is now locked up not only by the others but in his very self. Laing echoes this:

> The whole of our present civilization may be in captivity ... Man does not always need bars for cages. Ideas can be cages too. Doors are being opened in mental hospitals as chemical constraints become more effective. The doors to our minds are the most difficult to open.[152]

### (iv) THE TOTAL SOCIAL WORLD SYSTEM

The Dialectics of Liberation Conference, held in London in July 1967, was organized by the "anti-psychiatrists", Laing, Cooper, Berke and Redler. These "anti-psychiatrists" who had been working

Laing writes in *The Divided Self* (p. 25): "The greatest psychopathologist has been Freud." Freud was a hero "who descended to the underworld and met stark terrors there... We who follow Freud have the benefit of the knowledge he brought back with him and conveyed to us".

150. Laing and Cooper, *Reason and Violence*, pp. 113-14.
151. Ibid., p. 176.
152. Laing, *The Politics of the Family*, pp. 57-58.

on the study of families and scapegoating, saw these very processes as relating to certain political processes, in particular the Vietnam War, where the "enemy" (Them) earned certain negative attributions from Us. Violence existed at all levels; the conference, according to Cooper, was devoted to discussion about "mass suicide and mass murder and we have to achieve a minimal clarity about the 'mechanisms' by which these processes operate before we can talk about liberation". In fact, the analysis of destruction was the central concern of the conference and the contributions of Laing and Cooper were about destruction "by illusion and mystification".[153] The importance of the demystifying element is made clear in Laing's contribution, "The Obvious", which Cooper placed first in the book of conference papers. "The obvious is literally that which stands in one's way, in front of or over against oneself. One has to begin by recognizing that it exists for oneself."[154] Long concerned with unravelling deceptive and mystifying structures of experience and behaviour, Laing had ventured into a still more "macro-" context, the "Total Social World System".[155]

Does this mean he had taken a "political" stand on the side of the Left? During the 1960s he was increasingly identified with the Left. Sedgwick writes that around 1960 the then editor of *New Left Review* had assured him that "R.D. Laing is one of us". Indeed, Sedgwick writes, "for many years afterwards those of us who read New Left journals in Britain" were given the same impression.[156] Underground newspapers included articles and interviews with and about Laing and his colleagues. Laing was associated with the "sigma" project, which had preceded the underground[157] and Kingsley Hall was a scene of underground activity.[158] Sedgwick himself had written in his *Salmagundi* article on Laing, published in early 1971, that Laing had turned to "social radicalism"

153. Cooper, *The Dialectics of Liberation*, pp. 7-9. It should be noted here that Laing himself would certainly not accept the appelation "anti-psychiatrist" now if he ever did. Nonetheless it is a useful term to connote the work of Laing and his colleagues which directly challenges the paradigms of mainstream psychiatry, particularly in its non-analytic practice. Further it would be mistaken to see Laing and his colleauges as sharing a worldview in common. For example a major reason for Laing's break with Cooper was Laing's intense dislike of Cooper's brand of political activism and analysis.
154. Laing, "The Obvious", pp. 13-14.
155. Ibid., p. 15.
156. P. Sedgwick, "Peter Sedgwick Meditates on the Acceptability of R.D. Laing", *Listener*.
157. J. Nuttall, *Bomb Culture*.
158. Gordon, "Who is Mad, Who is Sane?"

and was a "left-wing critic".[159] Interestingly in the Penguin publication of this article, he adds a postscript accusing Laing of "betrayal" of his former "political and social commitment".[160] Contrary to his former position, in a later article in *The Listener* he even denies that Laing was *ever* left wing, or had any left associations! With a not too muted anger (and denial!) Sedgwick writes;

> ... as a member of the International Socialists since the late fifties, I knew who was around for serious political work and R.D. Laing was not only unavailable: he wasn't around anywhere, not even in the small back-room where revolutionary theory does sometimes have to be hammered out.[161]

Until recently though, Laing had duped them all—including Sedgwick. Everybody still wants to hang on to "their Ronnie".

Perhaps the explanation is that the Left had adopted Ronnie and not vice versa. Laing has himself said:

> I was never *political* in an activist sense. I suppose when people think of me as political, they're thinking mainly of the Dialectics of Liberation Congress. I guess I identified myself by being there, but even at the time I made it clear that I really had no idea what could really come of such an extraordinary conglomeration of people. Politically, I think I'm neutral really. I engage in no strictly *political* actions—except in the sense of following the *TAO*.[162]

In the same conversation he later said: "Of course I'm in favour of revolution. But I don't consider it a revolution when Tweedledum takes over from Tweedledee under whatever name he happens to go." This was perhaps an allusion to his being put off by the violence of some of the speakers at the Dialectrics of Liberation Congress, especially Stokely Carmichael.[163] The foregoing remarks were made in 1971 in what may be called Laing's transcendental period. There seems to be some denial on the part of Laing of his politics, such as they were. After all, he was not merely at the congress, his home was the centre for its organization.

However there is much truth in Laing's above assessment of his position. Laing said that he was

> "not an activist in the ordinary sense of the word". "Living in England", he observed, "made radical activism less pressing than in America". Besides, he felt that he was "temperamentally not very well suited for it".

159. P. Sedgwick, "Self, Symptom and Society" in R. Boyers and R. Orrill (eds.) *Laing and Anti-Psychiatry*. (Originally *Salmagundi* 16.)
160. Ibid., pp. 46-47.
161. Sedgwick in *Listener*, p. 646.
162. Mezan, p. 165.
163. Ibid.

> His own energies are devoted to what he calls "microrevolutions", profound changes in individuals, families, hospitals and other small institutions. These changes may in turn bring about others, not through dramatic confrontation but by personal contact. Kingsley Hall, it is clear, is one such microrevolution.[164]

This should be contrasted however with his 1971 statement: "As for Kingsley Hall I undertook that with many reservations, almost against my better judgement. I'm not sorry about it at all, but if I were to do it again, it would be something quite different."[165] To take the evidence on face value an ambivalence of Laing towards politics might be seen. But on another level, perhaps an explanation is that politics and other activity for Laing provides and has provided outlets for what is his basic personal purpose: *demystification and disillusionment, providing a translucent intelligibility to situations, to understand the order of things*. While his work may be *used* by people who want change, for Laing actual change is secondary. Thus he may participate in politics as a relatively marginal activity.

Laing has steered his own personal path which at times coincided with Left politics. Somewhat elusive and aloof, he had never committed himself to an ideology nor indeed to his "followers", keeping his distance from most. Much of his writing, particularly in *The Politics of Experience* can be interpreted in a number of ways—when he states a proposition, he often puts so many reservations to it that it could be construed as close to a denial. Laing was both in politics and out of them. There *could* be important biochemical factors operating in schizophrenia, but it is normally assumed by him that there are not. Control groups are irrelevant to his studies in *Sanity, Madness and the Family*, but comparisons with "normal" controls were in fact begun. And so on. Sedgwick writes that Laing

> had made a number of promises—or hints and gambits which were heard as promises—which obviously couldn't all be kept. He was balancing the revolutionaries with one hand, the acid-freaks with the other, the social workers, with one of his feet; and that only left his nose for anything else, if he was to keep any contact with the ground. All that plus his patients and literary friends—the dear, dear people who know him as "Ronnie".[166]

Laing occupies a sort of "half-in, half out position". This position, though, illuminates the fact that Laing is not primarily a political thinker—at least in anything like the accepted sense. His interest is in

164. Gordon, p. 61.
165. Mezan, p. 116.
166. Sedgwick in *Listener*, p. 648.

removing illusions so that we can understand what is going on. Doing something about it is a different question. Laing has had an abiding interest in the nature of rationality. When the context has broadened to the total social world system which incorporates the many sub-systems, contextually, metacontextually, and so on, "there is no further *social* context to which one can refer the intelligibility of the total social world system".[167] This system

> appears to be dangerously out of the control of the sub-systems or sub-contexts that comprise it. We seem to arrive at an empirical limit which itself appears to be without obvious intelligibility, and beyond this limiting context we do not know what further context there may be that may help us to set the total social world system in a larger pattern or design in which it finds its rationality.[168]

Laing says that in the total social world system there are some components which "do seem to be more irremediably irrational than others". Putting the end itself in brackets, "an action will be regarded as irrational if it is ostensibly a means towards an end, such that this means leads to an end it purports to avoid".[169] Such irrationalities in fact abound to a far greater extent than Laing seems to realize. However, he is interested in the "normal" or "hypernormal" situation to which far too little emphasis is given, at least in psychology.[170] The normal situation is where atrocities are eagerly and actively perpetrated, whether on a macro-level (as in many people feeling guilty "if they don't manufacture, deliver or drop napalm, etc.")[171] or on a micro-level (mother showing she loves her baby by her holding him out of a sixth-storey window and not dropping him—"the *normal* way parents get their children to love them is to terrorize them").[172] These perversions are commonplace and are the results of a "multi-generational spiral"[173] of misapprehension and projection.

There are

> amazing collective paranoid projective systems that operate on large scales. We attribute to them exactly what we are doing to them. Because

167. Laing, "The Obvious", p. 15.
168. Ibid., p. 16.
169. Ibid., p. 20.
170. Ibid., p. 27.
171. Ibid., p. 25.
172. Ibid., p. 27.
173. Ibid., p. 28.

we are seeing ourselves in them, but we do not know that we are. We think that they are them, but they are actually us.[174]

Each system has its elective focus.[175] Given this focus, be they mental patients or Vietnamese, it is then possible to act in "their best interests" with sincerity and concern. The more patients protest the less insight they display into their condition. The more concerned doctors become, the more "treatment" they need such as tranquilization.[176] Psychiatrists honestly feel they are giving people what they ask for: relief from suffering. This is but one example of the diametric irrationality of much of our social scene; the exact opposite is achieved to what is intended. Psychiatrists make fortunes by killing "souls". Mental patients have killed far fewer people than "legalized 'sane' members of our society".[177] Most people "will just do what they are told"[178] and feel guilty if they do not, "even if they think it is wrong". Indeed, we have a "reflex towards doing what we are told".[179]

We have then a situation in which people feel it is right to be obedient or, rather, wrong to be disobedient. Even those giving the orders may be mystified to the extent of believing what they are doing is right (such as psychiatrists). Whereas Laing would say that psychiatrists normally harm people, the psychiatrists (and many of the patients) would assert the contrary. For Laing this indicates the extent of their mystification. But their actions are often irrational means which achieve the opposite of what is intended. The problem is that too often they achieve what *is* intended—and it is the intention itself that is irrational. That is, Laing's definition of "healing" would be different from the mystified version that, according to Laing, most psychiatrists believe in. Their practice only avoids Laing's presumably demystified ends.

It may be argued that the total social world system and its mystifications and violence are intelligible not within a further context "beyond" this world, but in terms of concepts and movements which exist in the social system itself. The totality of the world may not be so perverted as to be univocally determined by the Us/Them dichotomy in which none of Us can possibly see that it is not Them that are "at fault" but Us. Demystification does not *per se* require a meta-context beyond the social system. Sometimes Laing recognizes

174. Ibid., pp. 28-29.
175. Ibid., p. 21.
176. Ibid., p. 18.
177. Ibid., p. 19.
178. Ibid., p.20.
179. Ibid., p. 32.

this: when he points to the dissonance between theory and practice, between ends and means, Laing writes that Freud demonstrated that "the ordinary person is a shrivelled, dessicated fragment of what a person can be".[180] "Normal" behaviour is the result of "repression, denial, splitting, projection, introjection, and other forms of destructive action on experience. It is radically estranged from the structure of being".[181] Psychotherapy as "an obstinate attempt to recover the wholeness of human being through the relationship between them",[182] could be one method of altering the situation of alienation. Obviously counter-cultural movements which aim at enriching and not destroying experience, as well as creating a new society in which the wholeness of human being could be achieved, are some kind of trends of possibility, even if seen as empirically impossible at present. As Sartre could point out, man, however alienated, is still man—he is never an object. In the introduction to *The Politics of Experience* Laing explicitly denies Marcuse's view that "dialectical theory finds its present truth in its own hopelessness".[183] In a review of *One-Dimensional Man*, Laing chides Marcuse for ignoring the Negroes' struggle in his analysis. "There is a *vicious* struggle within America, within and outside the universities and there are calls on physical as well as on moral and intellectual courage." Laing writes that Marcuse implicitly confesses his only hope to be in his own refutation and Laing comments, "And this will be accomplished, if at all, only by us, and only through our praxis".[184] This is one strain in Laing's political thinking.

The more dominant strain however is one that is a flow on from his earlier work and that of Sartre. Rationality cannot be found within the context of the total social world system in which we are imprisoned. The social system of groups *per se* violates the self. "To suffer society is enough", said Cooper. "Society is a concentration camp."[185] Laing avers: "We are all murderers and prostitutes—no matter to what culture, society, class, nation one belongs, no matter how normal, moral or mature one takes oneself to be".[186]

> Our alienation goes to the roots ... We are bemused and crazed creatures, strangers to our true selves, to one another, and to the spiritual and material world—made even from an ideal standpoint we can glimpse but

180. Laing, *The Politics of Experience*, p. 22.
181. Ibid., pp. 23-24.
182. Ibid., p. 45.
183. Ibid., p. 11.
184. Laing, "One-Dimensional Man".
185. Quoted in Nuttall, p. 222.
186. Laing, *The Politics of Expereince*, p. 121.

> cannot adopt. We are born into a world where alienation awaits us. We are potentially men but are in an alienated state, and this state is not simply a natural system. Alienation as our present destiny is achieved only by outrageous violence perpetrated by human beings on human beings.[187]

Alienation is induced too by the rigid dichotomy between behaviour and experience. "I cannot experience your experience" and vice versa. "We are both invisible men." I can only "experience you as experiencing", but you can only convey this through your behaviour.[188] Multiple spiralling into greater and greater disjunctions, or violent control of behaviour and even experience appears inevitable. Everybody in the world is rooted in alienation and, given "an ideal standpoint we can glimpse but cannot adopt", *social* liberation is impossible. Social man has stolen individual man's capacities. The violent scapegoating of Us and Them, which takes place on every level, has annulled human possibility. Men are "weighed down" by, among other things, "a sense that their very thoughts and feelings, in their most intimate interstices are the outcome, the resultant of processes which they undergo".[189] Each is from birth then at the mercy of the terror and violence of the others. A man can either alienate himself through mystifying himself and others or "he can also have what he does stolen from him by the agency of the others".[190] Either way there is no hope. Each is either serial other to the others or is caught in a nexus whereupon his experience is destroyed. Next to all this destructiveness the oft-quoted statement of Laing's: "Normal men have killed perhaps 100,000,000 of their fellow human beings in the last fifty years" seems to pale into insignificance![191] Those killed should perhaps have been thankful!

But no.

> Yet if nothing else, each time a new baby is born there is a possibility of reprieve. Each child is a new being, a potential prophet, a new spiritual prince, a new spark of light, precipitated into the outer darkness. Who are we to decide that it is hopeless?[192]

This seems in complete contradiction to Laing's earlier quoted remarks. If our experience is destroyed in a world defined by a man's

187. Ibid., p. 121.
188. Ibid., pp. 16-17.
189. Ibid., p. 25.
190. Ibid., p.25.
191. Ibid., p. 24.
192. Ibid., p. 26.

alienation from other men and his "possibilities" *qua* concept of "man", then this "spark" *is* hopeless. Laing cannot consistently hold to both positions. Where can "spiritual princes" come from if every man in the world is both murderer and prostitute and "educates children to lose themselves"?[193] In his chapter "Us and Them" Laing describes in more detail how the group destroys the individual, and groups create others for Them. At its conclusion Laing says that "We and Them must be transcended",[194] but everything preceding this denies this very possibility.

But perhaps this is denied only in the case of social liberation in the normal sense. Laing had corresponded with Timothy Leary and his co-workers about hallucinogenic drugs. "Laing visited them in 1964 and was impressed."[195] Not only was he interested in LSD,[196] but he also took an interest in Eastern religion and mysticism. The "inner/outer" distinctions had been questioned by Laing before, but Laing had not previously asserted that dreams and phantasies were just as real as the world of common sense. But he does in *The Politics of Experience*. Most people do not know that every night we enter zones of reality in which we forget our waking life as regularly as we forget our dreams when we awake. What are merely different modalities of experience are often labelled "'pathological' zones of hallucinations, phantasmagoric mirages, delusions. This state of affairs represents an almost unbelievable devastation of our experience."[197] "The condition of alienation, of being asleep, of being unconscious, of being out of one's mind is the condition of the normal man."[198] This being so liberation will take place only through an inner focus, opening up one's mind to experience. This can be done through LSD, Leary would assert[199] and Laing at times gives the impression that this is a way. "If I could turn you on, if I could drive you out of your wretched mind, if I could tell you, I would let you know."[200] But this can be interpreted not as LSD inspired, but as an elevation of "madness".

Maybe Laing was originally inspired by LSD (and the emphasis on entirely different modes of experiencing as legitimate) and saw certain "voyages of discovery" which LSD trips resembled as illuminating. "Madness may not be all breakdown. It may also be

193. Ibid., p. 24.
194. Ibid., p. 83.
195. Nuttall, p. 197.
196. See biographical note on Laing in Laing, *The Politics of Experience.*
197. Ibid., p. 23.
198. Ibid., p. 24.
199. T. Leary, *The Politics of Ecstasy.*
200. Laing, *The Politics of Experience*, p. 156.

breakthrough. It is potentially liberation and renewal as well as enslavement and existential death."[201] Indeed, "to be mad is not necessarily to be ill"[202] and the person entering the inner realm will find himself on a "journey".[203] Many become lost in the "foreign territory" of the "infinite reaches of inner space", but this journey or "voyage of discovery"[204] may be a "natural healing process" for some people who are labelled as schizophrenic.[205] Schizophrenics are in an excellent position to take this journey as their behaviour is "a special strategy to live in an unlivable situation".[206] That these people find the "normal" situation unlivable can mean an inducement to embark on a voyage. "Schizophrenics have more to teach psychiatrists about the inner world than psychiatrists their patients."[207] In fact "the secular psychotherapist is often in the rôle of the blind leading the half-blind". The label "schizophrenia" is not a pathological condition "but the label is a social fact and the social fact is a *political* event".[208] The schizophrenic who does *not* adapt to the normal alienated world may be less alienated than the normal. If he embarks on a voyage and returns, he may be a "prophet" or "a spiritual prince". They have dissolved their egos, journeyed and become saner. Indeed, future man "will see that what we call 'schizophrenia' was one of the forms in which, often through quite ordinary people, the light began to break through the cracks in our all-too-closed minds". Those schizophrenics who have gone and come back to us should be accorded "no less respect than the often no less lost explorers of the Renaissance".[209]

The liberated people then are those who have explored the "other world", who have seen the "light", who have had the transcendental experiences "which sometimes break through in psychosis"[210] (although Laing says that he is *not* saying that "psychotic experience contains this element more manifestly than sane experience".[211] Perahps he is here referring to Eastern mysticism.) Laing writes that "the light that illumines the madman is an unearthly light... He may be irradiated by light from other worlds". There should be some

201. Ibid., p. 110.
202. Ibid., p. 113.
203. Ibid., p. 104.
204. Ibid., p. 97.
205. Ibid., p. 105.
206. Ibid., p. 95.
207. Ibid., p. 97.
208. Ibid., p. 100.
209. Ibid., p. 107.
210. Ibid., p. 158.
211. Ibid., p. 112.

physicians and priests "who are guides, who can educt persons from this world and induct them into the other".[212] The only aim of the Philadelphia Association which was designed by Laing and his "anti-psychiatrist" colleagues to help schizophrenics, was Laing said, "to reveal the greater glory of God".[213]

It can be seen that Laing's interest has become mystical in this phase. There is no real division between his focus on the total social world system and on transcendence. The total social world system is viewed as an alienated unity ruled by a web of internalized and externalized violence which is spiralling towards final self-destruction. The only hope lies in finding an intelligible metacontext to situate this total context. Schizophrenic priests may show the way towards the Light. The barren, disembodied and terrifying world of the schizophrenic of *The Divided Self* has become that of society itself. The schizophrenic now can lead "normals" into "other worlds". Previously, normals, in the form of sane psychoanalytically-oriented psychotherapists, led schizophrenics out of the terrors of constant threat to a precariously balanced personal integrity into a communal world where relationship is possible. Schizophrenics moved from dark dungeons towards the light—in *The Divided Self* the schizophrenic does not see it and the psychiatrist does: in *The Politics of Experience* the schizophrenic can see it and the psychiatrist cannot.

Sedgwick in his original article in *Salmagundi*, realized that Laing had taken a mystical turn for the worse, but noted that "I do not believe that Laing's mysticism can run very deep".[214] He corrects this in the Penguin edition of his article with a footnote saying that he was wrong in this judgment. Why Sedgwick and so many others had refused to see Laing's *basic* mysticism in *The Politics of Experience* would be of interest. Perhaps it was because of the sympathy with Laing's work on the questions of the social settings of sanity and insanity and his interest in treating people as people. Even now Laing is the only psychiatrist so many people have read, and in English-speaking countries at least, he and his colleagues are almost the only psychiatric figures referred to on the general Left with admiration.

Of course, two strains in Laing's "politics" referred to above—the this-worldly and the other-worldly—are conflated by Laing, and it is normally not clear to which he is referring. People read into it what

212. Ibid., p. 115.
213. Quoted in Nuttall, p. 221.
214. Sedgwick, "Self, Symptom and Society", p. 43.

they liked. It is useful to revert to Sedgwick's statement about how Laing was balancing contradictory forces with all parts of his body—all claiming Laing as their own.

> The burden must have been insupportable; and one cannot blame him for doing what he did. For last year (1971) Laing dropped everything, dropped the whole lot and took off. He went to a monastery in central Ceylon to engage in a lengthy task of Theravda Buddhist meditation... Laing could not have gone on keeping everybody happy. In particular, he had to begin annoying either the revolutionaries on the left or the mystics and the transcendentalists on the somewhere else, at any rate not on the left...[215]

Laing's focus has moved from the system he is leaving to the system of mysticism. As was noted above already in his focus on the social world as an alienated unity of Us and Them in conflict, he has become a transcendental mystic.

## (v) TRANSCENDENCE

> ... in *Self and Others* there's a preface, a quotation I took from Confucius: "The way out is via the door. Why is it that no one will use this method?". Well that door has always been a revolving door for me. When I wrote that, I was aware of all this—that distinctions like self and other were peculiar constructions of the mind.—**Laing**[216]

Man in the Jungian mythos was always with his shadowy other self.[217] For Laing now, man, the shadowy other, the world itself are the scene, not of irresolvable contradiction, but of fundamentally limited vision. Bateson observed: "One of the things (the Zen Master) does is to hold a stick over the pupil's head and say fiercely: 'If you say this stick is real, I will strike you with it. If you say this stick is not real, I will strike you with it. If you don't say anything I will strike you with it.'"[218] This was formerly the scene of the double-bind violence for Laing. Now Laing sees it and similar modes as a means toward a transcendent Enlightenment. The wrong questions are posed in Western civilization which is tied up in knots. Taken on the phenomenal level, these knots are irresolvable. If I distinguish between I and You or real and unreal, I shall involve myself in an

215. Sedgwick in *Listener*.
216. Quoted in Mezan, p. 175.
217. Cf. The title of the English translation of Sartre's play, *Morts sans sépulture*, alludes to this theme, *Men Without Shadows*.
218. Cited in Mezan, p. 96.

unending spiral of destructive manoeuvres which make less and less sense and create a cumulatively greater disjunction or split. If I ask for a sense on this level, I will be answered with nonsense. But non-sense in non-sense. If I see the social world itself, not in its own alienating context, but in a metacontext which sees the fault in the common assumption of dichotomies as real, with the divisions of phantasy and reality, subject and object, as potentially within the bounds of sense, I may cease to look for sense itself in a predefined framework. Us and Them are not a projective splitting of mystification. The very distinctions can be resolved not dialectically into a unity which may go beyond them in an immanent sense, but can be seen as pointers to the mystifications of looking at things in *that* way.

Laing's *Knots* provide us with descriptive modes of what is normally seen as human bondage, but points to a context which entirely supersedes or transcends the former modes of looking at things, "... If it is not me, I am it, if I am not it, I am it, if I am it, I am not it".[219] "If I don't know I don't know, I think I know, if I don't know I know, I think I don't know."[220] Laing takes the consequences of contradictions such as these and finds them as leading to impossible situations within the terms of the context in which they are situated. Knots are everywhere, and everywhere irresolvable in earthly, rational or logical terms. Laing's *Knots* delve further and further into hopelessness in the usual way of looking at things. The more entangled one becomes, the less one sees one's entanglement and the less one can get out of it. Man has become so estranged from being that he does not see this estrangement nor the true reality. If one has not seen the gate to Nirvana, one may deny its existence. On the other hand, to talk in these terms is mystifying in itself since there is no gate through which one can walk.[221] "There is no way of knowing except to go through it."[222] This statement indicates that the question is meaningless in mystical terms. Laing says:

> It is heresy to say either that the world is real or that it is not real, or that the world both is and isn't real, or that the world is neither real nor not real. Saying any of those is likely to get you into a conflict that will produce anxiety that will produce shame that will produce guilt. You see, what we do is to impose on the *suchness* of things a duality, which sets up a conflict. Then we try to resolve the conflict by applying more dualities.

219. Laing, *Knots*, p. 47.
220. Ibid., p. 55.
221. Ibid., p. 85.
222. Ibid., p. 86.

It's like good and bad—when all I can do is feel good and bad—there's no room for anything else. It's the same for all these distinctions—heaven and earth, real and not real, existence and non-existence. You come to see the whole structure as the construction of the mind... And the thing about such questions is that I know they are unanswerable. But simply to tell you that isn't any good; so I try to help you to find out why you ask them.[223]

According to Laing,"the experience of illumination is not sudden, it's a gradual process of hard work and discipline", and he himself was engaged in "renunciation" which is "ridding yourself of attachments until you are maintaining yourself in a minimal fashion: you eat just enough, breathe just enough to stay alive, to continue". He was a vegetarian, slept little, got up early for two hours of yoga with friends at 7 a.m. until he left for Ceylon.[224]

What happens in the social world is "shadow" as in Plato's cave—and an interest in this distracts one from "illumination". What one chooses to do in this world is "a matter of indifference". For Laing, "the only guidelines from behaviour are not to hurt anyone, meaning not to cause harm to any part of the cosmos, and not to lie. Which you recognize is a very very subtle thing. I don't think I lie or do anyone any harm".[225] This was said in England. Sedgwick writes in a postscript to his article in the Penguin edition of *Laing and Anti-Psychiatry* that Laing's meditating in the middle of a civil war in Ceylon was like "a progressive cult-hero of the Thirties who decided to go off to a Catholic monastery at Burgos, behind Franco's lines, at the height of the Spanish Civil War. Withdrawal is not always a betrayal, but in this case what else is it?".[226]

In Ceylon, Laing meditated seventeen hours a day, and was regarded by the senior monk as doing much better than long-time experts in meditation. He did not plan to return to Europe, nor to write anything more—although, according to someone who has discussed this with Laing in Ceylon, if he ever wrote again it would be from the point of view of "meditation consummated".[227] Laing in this stage is involved in a personal project of illumination, of self-derealization. What of schizophrenia, sanity and embodiment? Laing had lost his preoccupation in psychiatry, but his attitude to schizophrenia is outlined in *The Politics of Experience and The Bird of Paradise*. It is one

223. Mezan, p. 174.
224. Ibid., p. 164.
225. Ibid., p. 164, 166.
226. Sedgwick, "Self, Symptom and Society", (Postscript Dec. 1971) p. 46.
227. Ibid., p. 46.

means toward Enlightenment. Obviously, those who cannot see through the knots in phenomenal existence are insane, and the further removed from this knowledge the less sane they are. But perhaps Laing would say that concepts of sanity and insanity are irrelevant insofar as one is referring to the social context. Anyone caught in the social context is mystified; perhaps it matters little which shadows the prisoners in the cave are seeing: the point is to see the total social world system as a prison. The body which in *The Divided Self* was the home of sanity, is now for Laing irrelevant, a shadow. "I understand that there are enlightened people who can return and occupy any *body* of experience they want; but I've never met one—if I have I didn't recognize him."[228] Presumably in Ceylon he met some such "person"—although his subsequent turning away from mysticism suggests disillusion with it.

The intrinsic meaninglessness of present human existence understood in human terms Laing shows at the conclusion of *Knots*. He takes a proposition "A finger points to the moon", puts it in brackets and says that the statement "A finger points to the moon is in brackets" is if bracketed and related to what is not bracketed as a finger is to the moon. If all possible expressions are put in brackets and all possible forms are then bracketed then what these are to what is expressionless and formless is as a finger points to the moon. But even the proposition "All forms point to the formless is formal". *Knots* finishes, not in futility because ultimately we can put everything in parenthesis and relate it to nothing at all, but in this:

What an interesting finger,
        let me suck it.
It's not an interesting finger,
        take it away.
The statement is pointless
The finger is speechless.[229]

Apart from the humorous and play aspect of this statement, what it means, Laing might say, cannot be explained. Nor can it even be *shown*. It must be *experienced*. The illumination itself will put the social world in a qualitatively different meta-context. As Laing puts it in *The Politics of Experience*, alienated man "does not know that where it all ends there it all begins".[230]

228. Mezan, p. 166.
229. Laing, *Knots*, pp. 87-91.
230. Laing, *The Politics of Experience*, p. 38.

## (vi) LAING'S JOURNEY

This chapter has attempted to trace a path.[231] Laing has moved far from the position in which the man who experiences the world as a prison without bars or a concentration camp without barbed wire needs to be freed from his imprisonment. At the time he believed this was to be done through sympathetic, humane psychotherapy in which a meaningful relationship—often the first one in the patent's life—may, with hard work, be established between two persons in a shared world of common sense. Laing's position underwent many metamorphoses as the contexts in which the "insane" situation occurred were in turn examined. As this happened, Laing's interest in psychoanalysis lessened, while his concern with interpersonal perception and group dynamics broadened. The schizophrenic was no longer seen as a fragmented person, living in a barren and terrifying private world, and who lacked the fulfilment provided by mature human encounter. In the false-self system of *The Divided Self*, the true self found a prison. Only by working through the dangerous and threatening situation in which the true self becomes more sure of its ontological foundations could sanity be achieved. The schizophrenic finds his strategems for living in an unlivable situation themselves insupportable. The therapist tries to provide a context in which it is no longer necessary for the schizophrenic to adopt these strategies of survival, and in which gradually, the schizophrenic may be able to find an alternative and a more gratifying way of living in the world.

Laing's search for an abiding rationality leads him through analysis of individual, interpersonal and familial situations to find the general world situation as still more irrational. Hope diminishes as the context widens. Finally the blatant or, as Laing might say, *obvious* madness of the social world and its subsystems leads to a withdrawal to a further meta-context—what Laing could term a sane schizoid position. But the position Laing actually achieves if seen in the categories of his early work is simply described as schizoid. Laing's journey has brought him full circle, but the points of arrival and departure may lead to a mutual questioning. Seen from the position of the point of departure (i.e. of *The Divided Self*), the point of arrival back is a schizoid condition. From the viewpoint of the

231. Laing's significant contributions to social intelligibility of "sick" situations are by no means dismissed: on the contrary, much of this chapter is devoted to a systematic exposition of certain of his insights. But the place of these insights and an evaluation of Laing's own situation are not the subject of *this* investigation. I have attempted an understanding of Laing's works in terms of *intellectual biography*. Perhaps this chapter raises the question with which it deals to a degree: "How is Laing possible?".

transcendental "withdrawn" point of arrival, the starting point of the journey is still very mystified and quite wrong—the schizoid has turned out to be right after all: society is a concentration camp.

Is it correct to ask which point is the right one? Looked at in individual psychological terms, perhaps the schizoid individual is insane. But the macro-political context is dangerous and mad as well. When the schizoid says that society is a concentration camp, he may express not only his own fear of relationship and dread of freedom—he may reflect something of the social context in which he lives.

Prefacing a case-study in *The Divided Self*, Laing quotes Sartre:

> I am not fond of the word psychological. There is no such thing as the psychological. Let us say that one can improve the biography of a person.[232]

Understood in this way, the purely psychological gives way to comprehension of the biography of a person which is political. This is not to say that the categories of psychoanalysis disappear. On the contrary they assume new dimensions in the study of man in society. To view individual disequilibrium solely in individual psychological terms ignores the social setting: to view individuals as the product of macro-political events is deficient in the opposite direction. Biography is an irreducible category.

As can be readily seen from this chapter, Laing's edifice finds many of its foundations in Sartre. Sartre has subjected his own condition to criticism. In *Words* he recalls how many of his own views were a product of his peculiar upbringing and his own personality. For example he wrote: "Mystified and a fraud to my very bones, I cheerfully wrote about our wretched lot."[233] Feeling impossible himself, he wrote that man was impossible. Spending much of his childhood in a room with his mother and without peers, he wrote of the imprisonment of man. Brought up by adults who accepted him not as a child but only as a miniature adult, Sartre was an impostor playing the roles expected of him. He found he had no true self: "Before my eyes, a jellyfish was striking against the glass of an aquarium, feebly gathering its ruffle and fraying in the shadows". He was "an empty palace of mirrors...".[234] He was the constant object of himself as other. He was dual[235] and goes so far as to ask whether what had happened in the past to "the person who bore my name"

232. Laing, *The Divided Self*, p. 120, quoted from Sartre, "Interview with Oliver Todd".
233. Sartre, *Words*, p. 156.
234. Ibid., p. 69.
235. Ibid., p. 136.

concerned him. Was he the same person in any sense at all?[236] Everything he did, once it was done was no longer his. The judgmental observer was always present, loathing the acts of what to others might appear the same person. There is a radical division between act and actor—Sartre as analyst never finds meaning in his act. His constant self-consciousness as other to himself is only matched by his hostility to himself. He judges everything he does harshly, loathing his own work, and is even his own witness for the prosecution.[237] Sartre writes of his condition:

> No one can forget me or pass me over in silence. I am a large manageable and terrible fetish. My consciousness is in fragments: all the better. Other consciousnesses have taken charge of me. They read *me* and I leap to their eyes; they talk about *me* and I am on everyone's lips, a universal and singular language; I have made myself a prospective interest for millions of glances. For anyone who knows how to like me, I am his most intimate disquiet: but if he wants to touch me, I draw aside and vanish: I exist nowhere but I *am*, at last! I am everywhere: a parasite on humanity, by my good deeds I prey on it and force it endlessly to revive my absence.[238]

Sartre's situation reads like that of the schizoids described by Laing in *The Divided Self.* In his chapter on "Self-Consciousness",[239] Laing describes the schizoid as "frequently tormented by the compulsive nature of his awareness of his own processes", by his "awareness of himself as an object of someone else's observation", and constantly under the eye of his own hostile self-scrutiny. There is "a constant dread and resentment at being turned into someone else's thing, of being penetrated by him, and a sense of being in someone else's power and control. Freedom then consists in being inaccessible." Freedom, for the schizoid, is not a positive freedom, but the negative freedom of elusion which finds its rationale in the danger others present to his very existence. The dilemma of such a person is that "he may *need* to be seen and recognized, in order to maintain his sense of realness and identity. Yet at the same time, the other represents a threat to his identity and reality". And this relates to his self-perceptions.

> Identification of the self with the phantasy of the person by whom one is seen may contribute decisively to the characteristics of the observing self... This observing self often kills and withers anything that is under its scrutiny. The individual has now a persecuting observer at the very core

236. Ibid., p. 149.
237. Ibid., pp. 148-49.
238. Ibid., p. 122.
239. Laing, *The Divided Self*, Ch. 7.

of his being.[241]

Above all else, at the same time closeness—especially loving closeness—threatens the schizoid's self.

If Sartre's *Words* calls into question the status of much of his philosophy—which, even without *Words* is evidently decidedly schizoid—Laing's development and views should be seen in the same light. Although Laing has recently taken a different path from Sartre (Sartre was a political activist of the extreme left while Laing disclaims significant political committment), Laing's views rest on the same problematic as Sartre's. This poses the question: was Laing's retreat to a monastery an illustration of bad faith or is it an instance of being true to oneself? Laing returned to England late in 1972, but his basic position remained the same for some time after.[241]

Harry Guntrip, a leading object-relations psychoanalytic theorist, writes of existentialism as finding human existence rooted in anxiety, despair, meaninglessness, triviality, futility and uncertainty that (and I quote this passage again):

> This surely is schizoid despair and loss of contact with the verities of emotional reality, rationalized into a philosophy; yet existentialist thinkers, unlike the logical positivists, are calling us to face and deal with these real problems of our human situation. It is a sign of the mental state of our age.[242]

Both Laing and Sartre are very popular. If their philosophies are schizoid, they have touched on the schizoid plight of millions. Fear of and inability to form authentic relationships, inner feelings of hopelessness, meaninglessness and futility, and the omnipresence of violence in subtle and not so subtle forms, together with a pervasive madness, seem to be part of the prevailing human condition. This may be pathological, but there is no apparent hope of cure.

Sartre takes a pessimistic and basically resigned attitude toward this situation. Laing finally withdraws from it altogether, perhaps still in search of a further meta-context in which to rationalize the madness of this world. Speaking of this prospect, Laing has said:

> Some people think that it may be possible to do this within a cosmic pattern. On the other hand, more than one person has said—and usually been regarded as mad for having said it—that perhaps God is not dead: perhaps God is Himself mad.[243]

240. Ibid., p. 117.
241. Laing, Interview in *Rolling Stone*. The introduction discusses the path he has taken recently.
242. Guntrip, *Schizoid Phenomena*, p. 48.
243. Laing, "The Obvious", p. 16.

# PART III

# CONCLUSIONS

# 6

# The Schizoid Problem Today

The world Sartre and Laing describe is primarily that of contemporary advanced Western capitalist industrial society—the first world—which may be considered schizoid.[1] The bureaucratic-technocratic communist second world seems for both Sartre and Laing to offer no hope for the salvation of man either: it seems bent merely on the perpetuation of its domination over the underlying populations which are in its sphere of influence, and on the acceptance of the status quo of the world balance of power through *détente* and the like. The third world appears victim to the first and, to a lesser extent, the second worlds, and seems to hold the only real hope for both Sartre and Laing: for Sartre through its political activity against imperialist aggression, and for the transcendental Laing through the way of life of meditation, yoga and contemplation. Neither Sartre nor Laing sees any hope in the Western world bringing the good life about, and it appears that they look to the third in desperation, since opposition in the first and second seems contained and containable in the foreseeable future.

It is important to note the place of the first and second worlds in the world as a whole: it would seem that it is these worlds which basically set the pace through their technical-bureaucratic apparatus. With the rapidity and systematic influence of advanced technological change, it may be seen that the fate of the world as a whole lies with what happens in the first and second worlds—they greatly affect the destiny of mankind as a whole.

The projects which dominate the world are those of Western man. Since communism is a relatively recent phenomenon, and the Cauca-

1. R. May, *Love and Will*, Ch. 1. Guntrip, *Psychoanalytic Theory*, Ch. 6. Guntrip, *Schizoid Phenomena*, p. 47. D. Cooper, *The Death of the Family*.

sian communist countries largely accept the Western capitalist conception of progress as advance in material production, it might be said that the project of the first and most countries of the second worlds lies in the continued pursuit of the logic of domination which has been that of Western man since the time of the first industrial revolution. The world Sartre and Laing depict is grossly affected by this, and in this chapter it is vital to note the systemic effects of this project on the entire world of mankind.

The chapter is principally concerned with the first world, but reference will be made to the second and the third worlds, to mankind as a whole who, because of immense technologization, has come increasingly to be one world. I am not concerned here about the schizoid problem in China for example—if there is one at all—but with that which pervades the dominant advanced capitalist technological societies, and through them to the influence on the world as a whole since the future of the world greatly involves the most powerful nations in it. It should be observed that the interest Sartre and Laing have in the third world is largely a reflection of their lack of hope in the first and second; and further this interest is not so much one which is optimistic that the third will prevail over the power of the first and second, but in a last-ditch stand against them. In the case of Sartre, the third world provides a witness to the ignominy of the first and second, and also the opportunity of recognizing itself in the victories and defeats that occur in confrontations. The third provides evidence of the power, courage and humanity of the victim rather than of an ability to destroy the executioners and bring about a transvaluation of values in an open and happy Promethean future for mankind as a whole. For Laing also the third world does not offer the chance of victory in the total social world system, and rather than struggle against the first and second worlds, he appears to view the only possibility of liberation as through transcendence of the social world itself.

The following attempts to formulate some explanations as to how we have reached the situations which Sartre and Laing describe and embody, for their work expresses some of the basic problems of our epoch, particularly that of the advanced capitalist societies.

These societies appear to have achieved a near all-pervasive integration of the schizoid problem on most of their levels. While my descriptions obviously involve differential responses on different strata in different societies, my point is that the schizoid *framework* is one which provides a base for the whole. I am certainly *not* saying that for example everyone in every society suffers severe schizoid depression but that the *problematic* most people live in these societies revolves around the schizoid problem so far as to call ours a schizoid era, in contrast with former depressive eras.

Many people in our society feel uninvolved, apathetic, cut off, withdrawn, split, discontinuous, afraid. It is a world characterized by a radical ontological insecurity, a failure of basic trust. Today most people find it almost impossible to trust themselves, other people or the general environment, for these do not seem sufficiently good and reliable. Paranoia seems ubiquitous, and sado-masochistic relationships seem to be the prevalent ones.[2] On all fronts the outside world seems to menace our very existence to the extent that genocide can be carried out by masses of "normal" people; where the human race itself has risked extermination through the agency of national leaders who would actually prefer us dead than red; and which now risks extinction through the abuse of nature and the population explosion. With the advent of the one world of the "global village", we are aware of the toll of human lives exacted this century not only through two world wars and the constantly present regional wars, but through the fascist and totalitarian regimes which exist and have existed in a large part of our world. Torture has reached epidemic proportions.[3] The constant intrusion and bombardment of social messages to conform that people receive from very early in life onward, militate strongly against individual feelings of freedom. People do not trust the outer world and withdraw, their false self systems maintaining the social facade, while their natural selves are seldom if ever brought to life. There is a nearly all-pervasive *fear* of relationship with the outer world—the environment is not seen as good enough to be trusted.

But can people then trust themselves? People are social, they need a facilitating environment and others for fulfilment of themselves.[4] Man has always been socially mediated. In the womb he is symbiotically merged with the mother. At birth he is almost entirely dependent on the mother who constitutes his world. He is dependent not only for the milk itself and the performance of elementary functions, but for his image of the constitution of relationship and "reality". The way the mother behaves towards the child is itself mediated culturally. Later the child's horizon expands to encompass father and siblings, peers, school, church and other broader social

2. A. Storr, *Human Destructiveness*, Ch. 3-4.
3. Amnesty International Report cited in the *Age* (Melbourne), 3 Dec. 1973.
4. E. Erikson, *Childhood and Society*, Chs. 1, 7, 11. E. Erikson, *Identity, Youth and Crisis*. Guntrip, *Psychoanalytic Theory*, Ch. 5. Winnicott, *The Maturational Processes and the Facilitating Environment: Studies in the Theory of Emotional Development*.

groupings. He learns to trust himself only through recognition by significant others, whereas a century ago in the West, this trust could be provided often enough since most accepted their station, duties and place in a world order, and the environment was in general predictable and reliable enough to allow some forms of personal identity to emerge. These can be described in Riesman's categories of "tradition-" and "inner-directed" man.[5] Freudian man's problems seemed to be Oedipal ones, and the individual had sufficient basic trust in himself and his environment to reach that stage. Those born in this century however, seem to have no fathers at all—or at least weak facsimiles of them. Traditional standards of authority seems to have crumbled, and people have become increasingly insecure at more and more primitive levels. While Freud's patients were hysterics, classical depression has largely given way today to schizoid depression.[6] While in past generations people had sufficient trust in themselves and their environment to make development to and beyond the Oedipal stage possible, this century has witnessed a *crisis of basic trust* in that firm ontological foundations are lacking—the schizoid problem is the dominant one.

The development from infantile dependence to mature dependence may be seen to be the largest problem in human life[7] but the incapacity to form any relationship at all in a free, spontaneous and unafraid way means that development beyond infantile dependence seems almost impossible for most. The fundamental problem is not the sexual one Freud found with his own patients. It is rather the problem of power and impotence in a continuous battle for recognition, although this is often disguised in sexual terms. There is a radical problem of *identity*, that of having any identity at all. The "other-directed", "one-dimensional" man is "ontologically insecure", afraid of his freedom, and is so split and withdrawn that he cannot recognize himself except through the view others have of him. He thus conforms, fits in, adjusts to the expectations of the social system he lives as his own. Seeing himself as nothing, the world is a maze of mirrors reflecting and refracting myriad images, none of which seems real. What is internalized from the external world is primary, but the external world itself consists among other things of his own projections. Modern man is lost in this hall of mirrors. He does not

5. D. Riesman; *The Lonely Crowd*: A Study of the *Changing American Character*, Ch. 1.
6. W.R.D. Fairbairn, "Schizoid Factors in the Personality" (1940) in his *Psychoanalytic Studies of the Personality*. Guntrip, *Schizoid Phenomena*, Ch. 1. May, *Love and Will*, Ch. 1.
7. Guntrip, *Psychoanalytic Theory*, pp. 148-49.

know where to go, or if he does, how to get there. Illusion and reality intermesh so basically that contemporary man is sure of little, and he is far surer of the "external" realities than of any "internal" ones. What are called "internal", "external", "real", "rational" and so on are culturally conditioned and relative.

Modern western man takes calculability and quantifiability as constitutive of rationality and reality. Development, for example, may be seen as increase in profits, Gross National Products, or technology. Achievement is seen in terms of reaching a high echelon in the business world and making a lot of money. Happiness is having a wife, two children, one's own house, a secure job (preferably with "prospects") and a television set. Meanwhile atrocities are carried out by such "normal" people in the third world. People have reflex actions to obey, to submit,[8] and this has been demonstrated with frightening ferocity in the experience of Nazism. The passivity with which the German population became the world's greatest murderers may be explained in terms of relations at the oral stage of development, as has been seen above.[9] Indeed it is the kind of fatherlessness Mitscherlich describes in which if the father is lost when the child vitally needs him to build up his own identity, he becomes entirely dependent on the mother for the rest of his life.[10] That is, he never develops autonomy and remains in a state of passive identification. This is what Horney entitles "the neurotic personality of our time"[11]—the lost, powerless, passive, empty and frightened ego that has dominated much of the world in this century. This is the schizoid world that Sartre and Laing both describe and confront. The way they describe the world is how so many people experience it themselves. This century seems to have been the one in which the most fundamental and rapid changes have been made in history. I shall try and come to terms with and understand some of the factors that have led to the radical alienation that Sartre and Laing describe and confront.

Man and his purposes and actions may be viewed *systemically*—as part of a larger system in which he inevitably lives. This may be described in terms of the variables of soma, ego, society (Erikson), individual, society, ecosystem (Bateson), or *umwelt*, *eigenwelt* and *mitwelt* (Heidegger). Man is irrevocably involved with all three variables, and within the system, change in one subsystem will have

8. Laing, "The Obvious".
9. *See* Ch. 4.
10. Mitscherlich, *Society Without the Father*, p. 258.
11. K. Horney, *The Neurotic Personality of Our Time*.

effects on the others. Thus, in acting in the world, man must recognize that what he does will not only have the effects he purposes (if it does at all), but will lead to alterations in the other subsystems. Over the past few centuries, man has used a "logic of domination"[12] in his dealings with the natural world, without counting on the side-effects of his actions. The result today is dramatically real in the possibility of ecocide. There are always "unintended consequences" of actions when action is not viewed systemically. Indeed it is absurd to assume that the consequences of actions will be what we will, where the actions have more than a minimal effect on the system as a whole. Freud had postulated his psychoanalysis as the third and greatest blow to man's narcissism, following those of Copernicus and Darwin.[13] These discoveries have helped to situate man, and should dispel the idea that man is not part of a system, that he is absolutely free and powerful. Thus, for example, the purposes of the hidden man behind conscious purposes need to be explored before we can properly understand what is going on. The net effect the grab-bag of individuals pursuing their own ends has on the social system and on the natural world, must be investigated. Further the effects of the contexts in which individuals and groups live have on activity and the nature with which they interact must be understood.

This century enacts such exponentially rapid change primarily through the medium of technology that it is impossible to calculate the unintended effects that have occurred in the various subsystems. The impact that man has had on his fellow man and the environment is enormous—so much so that we may see that urban man has created a second natural environment. Men who scarcely understand themselves unleash forces of which they know little on a world they understand only in terms of the particular interest of their speciality. They pursue individual or group ends without considering the ends themselves, or the consequences that the fulfilment of these ends will have on the rest of the world. For example, last century Western man decided that technology was good and ought to be developed as quickly as possible so that he could have "more". The result is that few seem to question the ends of development and want more and more of whatever happens to be offering—basically material goods no matter what their "use". The use men have made of technology has transformed the world—and with it man himself. Western man has become slave to the constitution of reality in terms of technical, instrumental or formal reason, which describes the real and the rational in easily quantifiable terms.

12. H. Marcuse, *One-Dimensional Man*, Ch. 6.
13. S. Freud, "One of the Difficulties of Psychoanalysis" (1917), in P. Rieff (ed.), *Sigmund Freud; Character and Culture*.

Technology which has been used blindly assumes such power that it blinds us to its oppressive use. Our relationships are always mediated technologically. Technology has become our ideology[14] and so far have we introjected this ideology that alternative ways of thinking are often literally unthinkable. This amazingly rapid technologization which has elevated means to often undisputed ends has brought such total change that the categories of power and impotence seem particularly relevant to human existence. Man now has such total power that he could destroy his entire world in a holocaust that could not be dreamed of a century ago. He is also totally impotent since he seems not to be able to control the movements of the monster he has created; he cannot control nature as his pure instrument; nor can he control the consequences to himself or the world of the enormous changes he has wrought. The system now seems to have a logic of its own, so alienated are we from what we do. "Determinism" seems to prevail since our "free will" seems virtually impotent. We seem to have relatively little control over our destinies, rather we seem progressively further enmeshed in the identity of a system which increasingly takes on a greater reality of its own while the individual knows himself less since he tends to feel he is or ought to be what is expected of him in his roles.

In this schizoid position there occurs a final unity of subject and object—the object has not been humanized, but the subject has been objectified so far that he sees himself as object and cannot conceive of himself as subject.[15] In this state of double alienation—alienation from his alienation—the subject is split into a collection of roles and is regarded as abnormal if he does not adjust to this state. This maladjustment might be a sign of independence, but is treated as failure thus bringing about a spiralling alienation of increasing intensity. It is not sick not to be able to live in an unlivable situation. On the contrary, the unlivable situation itself requires change.

This is the import of Laing's work which focusses on the contexts in which we live, and endeavours to view our lives systemically. Sartre too attempts to look at our lives in terms of the systems in which we live and finally explains our lives in ontological categories—those which are necessary to an understanding of our being. Both Sartre and Laing attempt to demystify our concrete

14. J. Habermas, "Technology and Science as 'Ideology'"in *Toward a Rational Society*.
15. *See* Marcuse, *One-Dimensional Man*.

situations in terms of the impact that an immensely powerful world he cannot control has on the individual. Sociological factors condition individual psychology. The development of both Sartre and Laing may be viewed in terms of their growing awareness of the immensity and dimensions of the contextual systems in which the individual finds himself.

For Sartre, man's freedom which was described as so shrivelled in his early work that it amounted to a freedom in chains, has virtually disappeared in his later work. The last vestige of self left to man—the possibility of refusal—has been taken away by a world which has finally closed in on him so far that intentions and actions are determined from outside and have a negative relation with each other. Sartre has drawn out the consequences of his early position by expanding the ontological prison of the self through the self and other to the group which assimilates the individual entirely—all that is left is the world of the imaginary. If Sartre's optimism had been the belief that we do not suffer for nothing, the world he describes in the *Critique* and afterwards makes even this "optimism" no longer viable. He has cured himself of his "illusions" but the "real" world is far worse.

Laing too has developed in terms of the appraisal of the effects that various contextual systems have on the individual and concludes that they have such an overwhelming effect that individual salvation is only possible through a mystical transcendence of this world which is a prison—this is what Sartre does with his world of art. If this is the only way out, it is because the individual simply does not count in our world: the group, the system, sociology are the centre of reference. Because people individually and collectively have so dramatically transformed the world during this century and at the same time dethroned God, the world appears more chaotic and out of control than ever. There is nothing firm to grasp. We are thrown into the world without recourse or excuse. We are alone and cannot control the consequences of what we do. Man is free, but is in fact manipulated by forces he cannot see and which he has himself set in motion. The outer world has an autonomy of its own in responding as a system to things individuals have done to upset the balance. There is an enormous feedback. The world system can be understood in the language of cybernetics as self-regulating or self-correcting, as the individual human being can be seen as homeostatic. But it can also be seen as a runaway system: conscious purpose scarcely figures in a world of so many hidden and dark forces.[16] The ego tries to

16. G. Bateson, *Steps to an Ecology of Mind*, Part IV.

adapt but is very weak, it has no power in comparison with the weight of the rest of the system. So far is man a part of the system that he can be understood only in its terms. A man is by and large his epoch because there is little space between individual and society. Biography however, deals not with a man in his context, but in his contexts. There is no simple division of man and society. As I have argued, there are many contexts—and these can best be understood in terms of contexts, meta-contexts, meta-meta-contexts and so on. Thus the cultural mediation of the individual is no simple matter.

The social context is a matter of many levels of mediation, a *hierarchy of contexts*. Thus for example the individual can be understood in terms of his early years in the family, which can be understood in terms of their upbringing and interactions with others and between themselves which requires still further analysis and so on. Also he can be understood in terms of his interactions with the social and natural environment past, present and future... To understand just one man entails an enormous complexity of intertwining networks, each having only a relative autonomy. Sartre's own massive work on Flaubert is such an attempt to account for the life of a man. When viewed systemically actions can be regarded in terms of "games" theory.[17] The individual, social and biological games we play with ourselves, others, and the environment which we try and manipulate, must be understood before it is possible to consider the possibility of our changing them.

Sartre and Laing have as a guiding theme a phenomenological approach to reality which does not rely on presuppositions, but rather brackets certain factors out of consideration during investigation. But as they proceed they bracket less and less out of their view, and the context becomes increasingly horrific. Relatively autonomous subsystems such as the family are found to be themselves part of other contexts such as religious systems, economic systems, educational systems, and political systems. The identity of a particular family is largly conditioned by the particular location it has in the intermeshing meta-contexts—and of course these in turn are conditioned by, and at the same time condition the contexts in which these meta-contexts are situated. In other words, the macro-system seems to be a particular combination of sub-systems, sub-sub-systems and so on.

Social theory has often tended to be either scientistic or positivist, regarding the given as value-neutral and unrelated to human interest, or it has tended towards holistic explanation regarding the totality as

17. T. Szasz, *The Myth of Mental Illness*, Part V.

basically determined by certain economic, religious or political factors. Both types of theory seem not to treat man as an intrinsic part of a system comprising a hierarchy of contextual subsystems which themselves are relatively self-regulating and autonomous. Both types of theory level facts—the positivists regarding all facts as equal and the holistic thinkers strait-jacketing the facts in terms of one or a small number of variables. Neither type can do justice to the incredible complexity of interweaving paths of individuals, systems, metasystems and so on. The whole, while not the sum of its parts is neither the product of them.

What has generally been ignored is the *generic* difference that a system has from its sub-systems. Cybernetically there is always another circuit required to explain a given system and another to explain the explanation and so on to infinity—a name is simply generically different from what is named. Thus, for example, certain Marxist theories would hold the bourgeoisie responsible for economic exploitation, and see in technology a simple capitalist manipulation for profit. This is seen without the effect of the technology created being considered. Rapid technologization was certainly begun in the interest of the expansion and development of production and profit, but this development, while it serves the large capitalist enterprises, must be seen not only as caused by it, but as having achieved a certain autonomy of its own, having its own logic and its own relation to other systems. Max Weber had foreseen the development of the world as an "iron cage" where bureaucratization, technologization and rationalization would produce "specialists without spirit, sensualists without heart; this nullity imagines that it has attained a level of civilization never before achieved",[18] This is a feature not only of capitalist societies, but of all industrially advanced countries, including the Soviet Union. This is the world Sartre and Laing express and endeavour to comprehend.

Both Sartre and Laing are essentially pessimistic. They both express the crisis of basic trust and the radical problem of identity in the schizoid world. Both attempt to come to grips with the problems and find no apparent solution. The world is out of control. Schizoid man is indeed technological man, who has so transformed himself and his world that he no longer has the means of recognizing himself. Everywhere there is fear and intrusiveness—there is no sense of authentic selfhood, of being a person in one's own right. On the contrary our identity is comprised of *not* being the outside world, and this, for Sartre, is our terrible freedom. We can see, but cannot act—

18. M. Weber, *The Protestant Ethic and the Rise of Capitalism*, p. 182.

we are in a prison without bars since there is nowhere we can go, nothing we can do which does not have paradoxical consequences. We are free for nothing. Others threaten us on all sides, and even where we unite with others, it is only against other people. Men are engulfed or fear they will be. They are mystified and do not understand what they are doing. They would like to have a meaning in their lives, but in their shut-in state this is impossible in a world of reversed finalities. These reversed finalities are the evil which pervades the world. Everything we do ends up being destructive. The possibility of good died with God. Scarcity, lack, privation, all imply evil; since there is never enough, we must fight to the death for food, recognition or control. The Other is always a threat to me—he always wishes to use me, objectify me, treat me as an instrument for his own ends. My anguish is me; were this to disappear, so would I. Freedom is never conceived of in positive terms since man as negativity simply can never be fulfilled—existence is privation which is the evil to which we are condemned. At bottom we are nothing, and it is *mauvaise foi* to think anything else.

Thus the schizoid position is the only authentic position for Sartre—the authentic man proudly lives his life sentence. The thin line between the world and myself must be preserved at all costs. My freedom is that I can preserve that, but, as I have observed above, even this is challenged as illusion in the later Sartre. The only way out is to keep one's own phantasy world separate and sealed off from others. The self as negativity described by Sartre is simply the classical existence-essence distinction reversed.[19] Thus the distinction between humans and the natural world is simply that the world *is* and the person *is not* the world. Therefore, there is nothing he *can be*.

Sartre's position is then a static one—it is a last-ditch defence against the would-be overwhelming forces of the outer world. It well illustrates Klein's paranoid-schizoid position for, on the one hand, the person fears being engulfed by the menacing others, while on the other, he feels entirely cut off from them and nothing inside himself. He is stripped naked only to find that he does not exist as anything. While this is inherently frustrating since he cannot reach himself, it also means that *they* cannot reach him either. Sisyphus can never be entirely taken over. The self Sartre describes can never be happy—it is condemned to be an empty hall of mirrors and will always be on the defensive against someone or something. This is his only way of knowing that he has an ego at all by finding its boundaries, by testing it against the intrusion of others. Politics is a polarization of

19. J. Wahl, *Philosophies of Existence*, p. 13.

oppressor and oppressed, but liberation cannot be promised since this would mean transcendence of the world in which we receive recognition. The sado-masochistic world of mutual devouring is the only world Sartre can envisage and there is no way in which there can be a development beyond it. This is certainly a sign of the times in that the amount of destructiveness that is present in the world is in fact, as enormous as Sartre contends. Sartre's world is our world, though we need not share his conclusions.

This is also the case with Laing—ontological security, a sense of autonomy and separateness in dialogic and free group relationships in which each person shares firm ontological foundations is not viable. The self has withdrawn as the threat to selfhood has increased. The love and beneficence proffered him by others is normally destructive to personal integrity. And evil again poses a universal threat—relationships are fraught with double binds. Laing sees this as connected with the social mess into which we have gotten ourselves through not knowing what we are doing, and putting ourselves into self-generating, degenerative depressive spirals which spell increasing destructiveness. We become increasingly afraid of others whom we need, the greater the fear, the greater the feeling of inner emptiness and the concomitant greater need for help from outside which generates still greater fear. We cannot start off by being ontologically secure because the world is not a secure place to be in—quite the contrary. This is the discovery Laing makes as he explores our contexts, meta-contexts and so on. The self disappears as the ground for security crumbles. The psychopathology of the individual gives way to the pathology of the human race itself today for which there is no cure. The individual's fright is quite justified: it is the self-certainty of the alienated conformity of other-directed individuals about the phantasms they see as reality that is for Laing pathological. The world, Laing avers, is clearly a terrifying and hostile place to be in. But there is no way out except personal transcendence of it to a meta-system which rationalizes this one.

But God is dead. This point is as important for Sartre as it is here for Laing. The consecrated mythology of the past is shattered. Sartre was born at the beginning of the century and spent his childhood practically fatherless, without his being treated as a person worthy of any trust at all. Nor could he believe in any foundation to his own family, nor in the theistic beliefs of his grandfather. Ceremony and ritual substituted for any form of conviction. For all intents and purposes, Sartre was a bastard since he had no feeling of belonging anywhere. The violent cataclysms of the two wars and the massive changes in the world that took place during this first half-century are witnessed by the bastard Sartre as a representative of man who felt himself to be without roots. The old patriarchal authority has crumbled, and people regressed to a more primitive position in which nothing could be taken for granted, everything seemed false and alien and there was a strong need for a new identity to be fashioned by people themselves. Yet there was nothing in themselves people could grasp, and at the same time the world was becoming increasingly technologized with the consequent specialization and greater alienation of people from themselves and others as they clung to their products to provide definitions for them. Technology became an ideology of its own and spun further out of control. Sartre found himself with a feeling of basic mistrust in a world reeling in opposite directions to the conscious purposes of many well-meaning people. Capitalists, while they obviously benefited from the mode of production, were also slaves to their own system. Workers who saw that they were exploited supported the Party and Stalinist Russia, neither of which offered an alternative life-style for the individual since, on joining the Party, the member had to leave his self behind; collective discipline and revolution seemed to demand in their adherents the very contrary of what the revolution was supposed to be about—human emancipation. Yet, without the selling of souls only individual solutions seemed possible. And here all that was left were gestures of defiance. Sartre could see his epoch bring to light so many truths about the human condition. The world seemed to be heading from one catastrophe to another—and there was nothing one could do about it without collaborating in the perpetration of these or other disasters. Sartre writes:

> Revolutions are now impossible. We are being threatened by the most idiotic and bloodiest of wars. The propertied classes are no longer quite sure of their rights, and the working class is losing ground. We are more aware of injustice than ever, and we have neither the means nor the will to rectify it. But the lightning process of science gives future centuries an obsessive presence; the future is here, more present than the present.[20]

Sartre sees our age as being judged as guilty by future men—but not by those presently living. He views our age as already dead and as alone in history.[21] There is no solution in the present—man is in complete solitude for the first time and sees himself and the world as *things*, about which he can do nothing. But modern man will be seen as guilty in future centuries—that is, if we were able to look at ourselves clearly, which we cannot, we should be aware of our guilt.

20. Sartre, *Saint Genet*, p. 598.
21. Ibid., pp. 598-99.

We could not bear to judge ourselves. What worse fate can there be than to be simultaneously *powerless and responsible*? This is what Franz sees in *Altona* and kills himself. Franz is "more unfortunate than a madman"[22]—the future which weighs so heavily upon him is the present he cannot bear to see. For Sartre the rest of us go on because we refuse to face up to the realities of the age. Demystification might mean the death of man, but without such revelation man is doomed anyway—if loser wins, the winner also loses. Man is a bastard—powerless, abandoned, thrown into a world he does not belong to and which does not belong to him. The bastard is schizoid man who is detached from himself and the world, neither of which is at all trustworthy. Life is a battle for survival, a series of roles and plays in an attempt to manufacture a sense of meaning. This is what Laing's journey is about too. The schizoid of *The Divided Self* finally sees that he is right after all—the only alternatives are playing at conforming which most people do without knowing it, or actually seeing the frightening reality which merits only mistrust. Neither alternative seems viable.

The world Sartre and Laing describe is that of Plato's allegory of the Cave,[23] but the cave is now the totality of the world itself. The sun is now black—God is dead. There is nowhere to go and the person who sees what is going on is an outsider who has no means of bringing salvation to his fellow men. There is no way in which these people will see that what they take to be reality is image and vice versa. Indeed they will not accept such deviant suggestions, and will accommodate persons making such suggestions under rubrics such as "mad" and "unrealistic". The Cave is a self-regulating system which accommodates alternatives to it under its own terms. Moreover, the modern cave is far more complex than Plato's: there is an enormous number of screens and mirrors—so many, in fact, that even the visionary is lost. There is no alternative reality and no way of righting this one. The world for Sartre and Laing is a vast prison in which the prisoners wittingly or unwittingly collaborate in the perpetuation of their servitude. The world and the men in it are hopelessly split and confused, each action seems doomed to backfire and worsen the fate of man in a self-generating spiral. The more he tries to reach some identity the further he becomes from it, and the more he needs it. The more he sees his plight, the greater the need and the less the means of

22. Sartre, *Altona*, p. 60.
23. Plato, *The Republic*, pp. 278-86. S. Doubrovsky, "Sartre and Camus: A Study in Incarceration", p. 92. E. Fromm in Fromm et al, *Zen Buddhism and Psychoanalysis*, p. 109. P. King, "Alienation and the Individual", *British Journal of Social and Clinical Psychology* 7, p. 83.

solving it. He becomes more desperate and finally more apathetic and cut off, and less able to deal with the problems of the day. The world is tied up in knots.

Can we accept the views of Sartre and Laing? How much are they a product of the alienated worlds they describe so despairingly?

I have suggested that the rapid rise of capitalism and the peculiar position of lightning technologization which embodied the project of western man of recent centuries which follows a logic of domination, has resulted in enormous changes in the world to such an extent that we live in a second natural environment. What has been neglected is the systemic nature of man. The schizoid split enshrined in occidental culture, both classical and modern, between mind and body, denoted the almost infinite power of mind and the subservient and instrumental nature of the body and the natural world which were to be the vehicles for the realization of the wishes of the mind. Western man, especially of late, has generally regarded the body and nature as objects to be dominated—the body has long been the subject of contempt for its "imperfections" and has generally been regarded as a prison. Western man has valued cerebration much over emotion[24] and his projects have been in accord with an intellectual rationality (latterly under the form of scientific calculability) rather than in relation to a realization of the self as a whole on earth—a Promethean vision.

Marx, particularly in his early works, focused on the concept of nature, where liberation in a communist society would be the solution to the riddles of history—human beings would no longer be aliented from nature which was man's "inorganic body", nor from each other, but would so transform man and nature that naturalism and humanism would coincide. This involved the transcendence of the capitalist system and ethic which meant that man lost himself in the labour he put into the production of commodities which became fetishes. There was an image of a truly human society to be found in an alienated form in the transcendentalism of Western philosophy which, for Marx, expressed itself most completely in Hegel's system. Man could realize his possibilities through the transformation of the world through practice. The answers to philosophical problems, according to Marx, were to be found in the transformation of the conditions in which these problems arose—the problems would disappear with the abandonment of the conditions which gave these problems such prominence. The need for God was testimony to the alienation of man. Salvation

24. Fromm in Fromm et al, pp. 108-9.

was to be earthly and was the demand for the transcendence of capitalist society. Yet Marx himself was bound to be affected by the natural scientific approach of thc rising bourgeoisie which saw salvation in the development of production. If there is a growing ambiguity in Marx himself in regard to the linear development of natural science and the primary importance of the economics of who owns what, this was far greater in Engels and many of the Marxist theorists who followed him. These seemed to accept the logic of domination encapsulated in the approach of nineteenth century natural science—but it was the working class which was to profit, not the capitalists. There was thus an important positivist stream in Marxism.[25]

Yet the influence that rapid technologization was to have on man himself and the world he lived in, was largely unaccounted for in Marxism. As with many non-Marxist thinkers, Marxists saw technology as liberating so long as it was in the right hands—Lenin even saw Communism as Socialism plus electricity! Marxists, along with other materialists killed God and substituted economic salvation. The scientific attack on the resources of nature and of man was well under way at the beginning of this century, but little damage seemed to have been done. However, with an exponentially expanding technology bent on domination and delivering the goods, the impact on the world on all levels was enormous—from the inner dimensions of man himself, through to the thoughtless plundering of the natural. The world was changing drastically, and people felt a great need to find a secure identity for themselves. But God had been killed, and all that was left was what technology could offer. Twenthieth century technology provided not only a greater range and number of material goods, but the means of destroying mankind itself physically through nuclear bombs and psychologically through, for example, the mass media. People felt less and less whole as specialization, rationalization and bureaucratization placed people in boxes, and divided them still further into parts and roles. The amount of destructiveness of this century is truly monstrous on all levels.

With the impact of unplanned and largely capitalist technology on the world came gross systemic feedback. Before this century nature was generally untouched, and people's lives had a general stability about them—even where there was much misery. The abreactions to man's practice were not so very great, and could be largely accommodated. However, the impact of the monentous transformations

25. A. Schmidt, *The Concept of Nature in Marx.*

this century have had large repercussions throughout all systems. Technology has now become the dominant ideology, and people view their lives in terms of the expectations of the technical social system. Man is far more divorced from his actions than previously, simply because these actions have far larger import across the board. People do not feel that the technical system they live is theirs, but so far has it entered men's souls that life without it is largely inconceivable. Man is more manipulated than ever and has fewer means to do anything about it, since the technological system which he created and lives has achieved an autonomous existence of its own in terms of the "unintended consequences" of technological activity.

The world is near ecological disaster—a "paradoxical" consequence of thoughtless technologization aimed at "development", rather than its being regarded as a systemic *part* of the world-system with repercussions for the whole. Thus while bureaucratic technological capitalism and "socialism" seem to deliver the goods, the people who receive them are almost totally alienated from themselves, their society and the natural world. The universal pathology in modern civilization is schizoid depression which is a reflection and expression of the larger schizoid world people reproduce, and which is reproduced in them. Often people look inside themselves to find nothing except what has been done to them. In this situation, Sartre's affirmation of man as "nothingness" makes sense as does Laing's insistence on contextually situating the person making extreme situations an expression of the norm and incapable of solution. The age of "psychological man" that Phillip Rieff announces [26] is, in fact, one of primary ontological insecurity—it is the anxiety of the schizoid problem.

Is there a solution? Perhaps the psycho-sociology of Sartre and Laing need not be entirely accepted, for what they seem to emphasize above all is the effect the systems have on us. Sartre looks at the paradox of intention and consequence while accepting the schizoid premise that a man is only consciousness and that is nothingness. Later he finds that a man is under the total control of pledged and serial groups, again not taking sufficient account of the fact that an individual not only can belong to several groups at once, some of which conflict with each other in some areas thus leaving a little space for individual action, but also that, while a man is constituted, he is also constituting. There is a two-way relation between

26. P. Rieff, *Freud: the Mind of the Moralist*, Ch. 10. See also *Psychological Man: Approaches to an Emergent Social Type*, *Salmagundi* 20, especially the contribution of M. Beldoch, "The Therapeutic as Narcissist".

a man and his group—although in the case of a man who feels he is nothing, there seems to be influence in only one direction. In Laing too, there is this same impotence—the contexts, meta-contexts and contexts tend to look as though there is only a one-way influence on the individual.

The systems seem always to have autonomies of their own. For example, while in *The Divided Self*, Laing's patients sometimes talk schizophrenese and can reach some form of integration and basic trust, in *Sanity, Madness and the Family*, the schizophrenic member of the family scarcely seems to take part, or exert any influence whatever on the rest of the family. Finally in *Knots*, the schizophrenic's only way out is through a mystical transcendence. The man who is nothing can have no effect on his fellow man which cannot be entirely co-opted by the existing established systems. Yet the influence of such people as Sartre and Laing has exerted *some* influence in established societies—not an enormous amount, much less an amount which would actually encourage fundamental change in social structures.

Certainly, the analyses of Sartre and Laing do not point in the direction of revolution—or even in the direction of a more humane society. But one way of making their theories true is for a lot of people to accept them entirely—that is not to try and exert individual and collective influence on the established systems, subsystems, other individuals and themselves. Our method of analysis need not be theirs—*daseinsanalyse* and the English object-relations school could be more viable psychologies than Sartre's and the "non-psychology" of the later Laing. Man is not nothingness; it is true however that he often *feels* himself to be so, and it is the role of humanistic psychotherapy among other things to help the individual disclose this to himself and feel more ontologically secure, to feel more as a person instead of desperately attempting to *appear* to himself and others that he is one. The power or impotence, all or nothing, active or passive dichotomies certainly inform pathological relationships, particularly of the early oral kind. But it is not *necessary* to accept this framework. Man, as Sartre himself points out, is always man no matter how alienated his practice is. It may be possible to transcend the schizoid stage of development on micro-levels through not accepting their final necessity.

As I suggested in the Introduction, Sartre and Laing have a basically schizoid view of what it is to be a person or self. Relationships are viewed in terms of persecution, theft and intrusiveness and the only ultimate alternatives are isolation and fusion. The self is split off from the body and the world and individuality is constituted outside relationship for otherwise one would be swallowed up by others. Destructiveness for Sartre and Laing is located always outside the self, suggesting that there is a good deal of projection operating. The inner world of hostile object-relations is transposed to the hostile aspects of the outer world which themselves provide feedback for introjection and vice versa. Persecutory anxiety is not seen by Sartre and Laing as an intrinsic part of the dynamic self in early object-relations, but the external world of others instead is seen as inherently persecutory. Further this split of the object into its good and bad aspects which are seen as far apart from each other may lead to an idealized view of what a self is as a safeguard against the fear of persecution[27] A framework which is not schizoid might well view the self in an integrated way in which both good and bad aspects find their place together in a situation in which the good aspects are usually sufficiently strong to accept the existence of the bad aspects within the self and to resist their onslaughts. This by no means implies that the outer world is good, but rather that the self becomes strong enough to cope with the demands of life in an alienated world.

But what of the macro-levels of this world? It would seem from my argument that men are enmeshed in a large number of very complex contextual systems. It is decisive to unravel and understand the workings of the systems we live. We could not lose by doing so, and it might be possible to confront and effect some changes which would be important. If we do not try and understand man systemically and take some decisive action, then the human race is doomed to keep careering out of control in its activities, since these have such large systemic effects. The failure of basic trust today in this schizoid world involves a *fear* of trusting ourselves and others. Much of this fear is often justified since the world is a frightening place. But it is not *only* a frightening place and many schizoid fears are not justified. Indeed when people learn early that nothing is trustworthy, they invariably begin to treat themselves and others as if they were not trustworthy—which makes the world a still more frightening place, and they feel themselves to be still more bad or empty. It is important that we learn to trust in ourselves and in the social environment that which merits trust and to mistrust that which does not. This involves transcending the all or nothing schizoid framework, and daring to look at ourselves and the world realistically. The overcoming of basic fear of relationship and involvement is a pre-requisite for any human progress. While the world today is a schizoid one, it will

27. *See* Melanie Klein; "Notes on Some Schizoid Mechanisms" in Joan Riviere (ed.), *Developments in Psychoanalysis*.

only be possible to transform it in any way by not accepting its categories as finally valid. However, much work needs to be done to illuminate the workings of man and his world today, particularly in the areas of drawing out the consequences of psycho-sociological theory.

The world Sartre and Laing describe is one where our worst fears are justified. What is required is that we do not accept this picture as finally true, but as one that we *fear* might be finally true. I do not believe that it depicts anything ontologically inherent in the human situation as such, but results from men's socio-historical practice. In order to change this picture which appears an appropriate one to so many, a thoroughgoing transformation of the world which requires such ways of seeing is necessary.

# BIBLIOGRAPHY AND INDEX

# Bibliography

Works are cited in full only in the Bibliography. Footnote references are given by the simple citation of author and full title of the work for the first reference, followed by the author's surname and a shortened version of the title (where necessary) for subsequent references.

The Bibliography is arranged in alphabetical order of authors' surnames and of titles of works by the same author except in the cases of Sartre and Laing. As Sartre and Laing are the major authors under consideration, their works are cited in chronological order of first publication.


Almond, G.A. *The Appeals of Communism*, Princeton University Press, New Jersey, 1954.

Aron, R. *Marxism and the Existentialists*, Simon and Schuster, New York, 1970.

———. *The Opium of the Intellectuals*, W.W. Norton, New York, 1962.

*Australian and New Zealand Journal of Psychiatry*, IV, 4, 1970.

Barnes, M. and Berke, J. *Mary Barnes: Two Accounts of a Journey Through Madness*, MacGibbon and Kee, London, 1971.

Bateson, G. *Steps to an Ecology of Mind*, Paladin, Frogmore, 1973.

Bateson, G., Jackson, D.D., Haley, J. and Weakland, J. "Toward a Theory of Schizophrenia", *Behavioral Science*, I, 1956.

de Beauvoir, S. *Force of Circumstance*, tr. R. Howard, Penguin Books, Harmondsworth, 1968.

———. "Jean-Paul Sartre: Strictly Personal", tr. M. Cowley, *Harper's Bazaar*, Jan. 1946.

———. *The Prime of Life*, tr. P. Green, Lancer Books, New York, 1962.

Bedloch, M. "The Therapeutic as Narcissist" in *Psychological Man: Approaches to an Emergent Social Type Salmagundi*, 20, Summer-Fall 1972.

Bergler, E. "Psychoanalysis of Writers and of Literary Productivity", *Psychoanalysis and the Social Sciences*, I, 1947.

Bettleheim, B. *The Informed Heart*, Paladin, London, 1970.

Boros, M.-D. *Un sequestre: l'homme sartrien*, Nizet, Paris, 1968.

Boss, M. *Psychoanalysis and Daseinsanalysis*, Basic Books, New York, 1963.
Burnier, M.-A.*Choice of Action*, tr. B. Murchland, Random House, New York, 1968.
Camus, A. *The Myth of Sisyphus and Other Essays*, Vintage Books, New York, 1955.
Caute, D. *Communism and the French Intellectuals: 1914-1960*, Andre Deutsch, London, 1964.
———.*The Fellow-Travellers*, Weidenfeld and Nelson, London, 1973.
Charlesworth M. *The Existentialists and Jean-Paul Sartre*, University of Queensland Press, Brisbane, 1975.
Chiaromonte, N. "Sartre and the Prize", *Encounter*, XXIV, Feb. 1965.
Contat, M and Rybalka, M, *Les Ecrits de Sartre*, Gallimard, Paris, 1970.
Cooper, D. *The Death of the Family*, Allen Lane, The Penguin Press, London, 1971.
———.(ed.) *The Dialectics of Liberation*, Penguin Books, Harmondsworth, 1968.
Cranston, M. *Sartre*, Barnes and Noble, New York, 1962.
———."Sartre and Violence", *Encounter*, XXIX, 1, July 1967.
Cumming, R. "The Literature of Extreme Situations" in M. Phillipson (ed.); *Aesthetics Today*, Meridian Books, Cleveland, 1961.
Doubrovsky, S. "Sartre and Camus: A Study in Incarceration", *Yale French Studies*, 25, Spring 1960.
Easton, L. and Guddat, K.H. (eds.) *Writings of the Young Marx on Philosophy and Society*, Doubleday, New York, 1970.
Erikson, E. *Childhood and Society* Penguin Books, Harmondsworth, 1965.
———."Identity and the Life Cycle", *Psychological Issues*, I, 1, 1959.
———.*Identity, Youth and Crisis* Faber and Faber, London, 1968.
Esterson, A. *The Leaves of Spring*, Penguin Books, Harmondsworth, 1972.
Fairbairn, W.R.D. "On the Nature and Aims of Psychoanalytical Treatment", *International Journal of Psychoanalysis*, 39, 1958.
———."Schizoid Factors in the Personality" (1940) in his *Psychoanalytic Studies of the Personality*, Tavistock, London, 1952.
Fell, J.P. "Sartre's *Words*: an Existential Self-Analysis", *Psychoanalytic Review*, 55, 3, 1968.
Friedenberg, E. *Laing*, Fontana Modern Masters, London, 1973.
Frued, S. "On Narcissism" (1914). "One of the Difficulties of Psychoanalysis" (1917) in P. Rieff (ed.) *Sigmund Freud: General Psychological Theory*, Collier Books, New York, 1963.
———."The Relation of the Poet to Daydreaming" (1908); "The Unconscious" (1915); "Reflections upon War and Death" (1915); "Why War?" (1932); in P. Rieff (ed.) *Sigmund Freud: Character and Culture*, Collier Books, New York, 1963.
Fromm, E. *The Fear of Freedom*, Routledge and Kegan Paul, London, 1960.
———.*et al. Zen Buddhism and Psycholanalysis*, Harper, New York, 1960.
Garaudy, R. "False Prophet: Jean-Paul Sartre" in G. Novack (ed.) *Existentialism Versus Marxism: Conflicting View of Humanism*, Delta Books, New York, 1966.

Gerth, H.H. and Mills, C. Wright (eds.) *From Max Weber: Essays in Sociology*, Oxford University Press, New York, 1958.

Glicksberg, C.I. *The Ironic Vision in Modern Literature*, Nijhoff, The Hague, 1969.

———.*The Tragic Vision in Twentieth Century Literature*, Southern Illinois University Press, Carbondale, 1963.

Goffman, E. *Asylums: Essays on the Social Situation of Mental Patients and Other Inmates*, Penguin Books, Harmondsworth, 1968.

Gordon, J.S. "Who is Mad? Who is Sane?", *Atlantic Monthly*, Jan. 1971.

Gorz, A. *The Traitor*, John Calder, London, 1960.

Graves, R. *The Greek Myths*, Penguin Books, Harmondsworth, 1960, Vol. I.

Guntrip, H. *Personality Structure and Human Interaction*, International Universities Press, New York, 1961.

———.*Psychoanalytic Theory. Therapy and the Self*, Basic Books, New York, 1971.

———.*Schizoid Phenomena, Object-Relations and the Self*, Hogarth Press, London, 1968.

Habermas, J. *Knowledge and Human Interest*, Heinemann, London, 1972.

———."Technology and Science as 'Ideology'" in his *Toward a Rational Society*, Beacon Press, Boston, 1970.

Horney, K. *The Neurotic Personality of Our Time* W.W. Norton, New York, 1937.

Jeanson, F. "Hell and Bastardy", *Yale French Studies* 30.

———. Idem. *Sartre par lui-même*, Editions du Seuil, Paris, 1955.

Jolivet, R. *Sartre ou la théologie de l'absurde*, Le Signe, Paris, 1965.

King, P. "Alienation and the Individual", *British Journal of Social and Clinical Psychology* 7, 1968.

Klein, M. "Notes on Some Schizoid Mechanisms" in J. Riviere (ed.) *Developments in Psychoanalysis*, The Hogarth Press, London, 1952.

Laing, R.D. (1957) "An Examination of Tillich's Theory of Anxiety and Neurosis", *British Journal of Medical Psychology*, XXX, p. 88 ff.

Laing, R.D. and Esterson, A. (1958) "The Collusive Function of Pairing in Analytic Groups", *British Journal of Medical Psychology*, XXXI, pp. 117-23.

Laing, R.D. (1960) *The Divided Self: An Existential Study in Sanity and Madness*, (Preface to Pelican Edition, 1965) Penguin Books, Harmondsworth, 1965.

———.(1961) *The Self and Others*, Tavistock, London.

———.(1962) "Series and Nexus in the Family", *New Left Review*, 15, May-June.

———.(1964) "One-Dimensional Man", *New Left Review*, Summer.

———.(1964) "Practice and Theory—The Present Situation", Sixth International Congress of Psychotherapy, *Psychother Psychosom*, 13, 58-67, 1965.

———.(1964) "What is Schizophrenia?", Paper read to the First International Congress of Social Psychiatry, *New Left Review*, 28.

Laing, R.D. and Cooper, D.G. (1964) *Reason and Violence: A Decade of Sartre's Philosophy, 1950-1960*, Tavistock, London.

Laing, R.D. and Esterson, A. (1964) *Sanity, Madness and the Family: Families of Schizophrenics* (Preface to Second Edition, 1969), Penguin Books, Harmondsworth, 1970.

Laing, R.D. (1965) "Mystification, Confusion and Conflict" in I. Boszormenyi-Nagy and J.L. Framo (eds.) *Intensive Family Therapy: Theoretical and Practical Aspects*, Harper and Row, New York.

Laing, R.D., Phillipson, H. and Lee, A.R. (1966) *Interpersonal Perception: A Theory and Method of Research*, Tavistock, London.

Laing, R.D. (1967) "Family and Individual Structure" in P. Lomas (ed.) *The Predicament of the Family*, Hogarth Press, London.

———.(1967) "The Obvious" in D. Cooper (ed.) *The Dialectics of Liberation*, Penguin Books, Harmondsworth, 1968.

———.(1967) *The Politics of Experience and The Bird of Paradise*, Penguin Books, Harmondsworth.

———.(1967) "The Study of Family and Social Contexts in Relation to the Origin of Schizophrenia" in J. Romano (ed.) *The Origins of Schizophrenia, Excerpta Medica*, International Congress Series 151, Amsterdam.

———.(1968) "Metanoia: Some Experiences at Kingsley Hall, London" in H.M. Ruitenbeek (ed.) *Going Crazy: The Radical Therapy of R.D. Laing and Others*, Bantam Books, New York, 1972.

———.(1969) *Self and Others*, Penguin Books, Harmondsworth, 1971.

———.(1970) *Knots*, Pantheon Books, New York.

———.(1971) *The Politics of the Family and Other Essays*, Tavistock, London.

———.(1971) Cited at length by P. Mezan, "After Freud and Jung, Now Comes R.D. Laing", *Esquire*, LXXVII, 1, Jan. 1972.

———.(1973) Interview in *Rolling Stone*, 142, August.

Laswell, H. *Psychopathology and Politics*, Viking Press, New York, 1960.

Leary, T. *The Politics of Ecstasy*, Paladin, London, 1970.

Lilar, S. *A propos de Sartre et de l'amour*, Grasset, Paris, 1967.

Marcuse, H. *One-Dimensional Man*, Beacon Press, Boston, 1964.

———."Sartre's Existentialism" in his *Studies in Critical Philosophy*, New Left Books, London, 1972.

Marx, K. *The Difference Between the Democratean and Epicurean Philosophy*, in N.D. Livergood, *Activity in Marx's Philosophy*, Nijhoff, The Hague, 1967.

Merleau-Ponty, M. *Sense and Non-Sense*, Northwestern University Press, Evanston, 1964.

Mezan, P. "After Freud and Jung, Now Comes R.D. Laing", *Esquire* LXXVII, 1, Jan. 1972.

Michel, L. and Sewall, R.B. (eds.) *Tragedy: Modern Essays in Criticism*, Prentice-Hall, New Jersey, 1963.

Mitscherlich, A. *Society Without the Father: A Contribution to Social Psychology*, Tavistock, London, 1969.

Molnar, T. *Sartre: Ideologue of Our Time*, Funk and Wagnalls, New York, 1968.

*Nation* (Editorial); "On the Need for Dialogue", CC, 19 April, 1965.
Plato, *The Republic*, Penguin Books, Harmondsworth, 1955.
Rieff, P. *Freud: The Mind of the Moralist*, Methuen, London, 1965.
Riesman, D. *The Lonely Crowd: A Study of The Changing American Character*, Yale University Press, New Haven, 1961.
Romano, J. (ed.) *The Origins of Schizophrenia, Excerpta Medica*, International Congress Series 151, Amsterdam 1967.
Ruitenbeek, H. (ed.) *Psychoanalysis and Existential Philosophy*, Dutton, New York, 1962.
Rycroft, C. *A Critical Dictionary of Psychoanalysis*, Penguin Books, Harmondsworth, 1972.
Sartre, J.-P. (1936) "Erostratus" in his *Intimacy*, tr. L. Alexander, Panther, London, 1960.
———.(1937) "The Wall" in *Intimacy*.
———.(1938) "Childhood of a Leader" in *Intimacy*.
———.(1938) "Intimacy" in *Intimacy*.
———.(1938) *Nausea* tr. R. Baldick, Penguin Books, Harmondsworth, 1965.
———.(1938) "The Room" in *Intimacy*.
———.(1939) *The Emotions: Outline of a Theory*, tr. B. Frechtman, Philosophical Library, New York, 1948.
———.(1943) *Being and Nothingness* tr. H.E. Barnes, Washington Square Press, New York, 1966.
———.(1943) *The Flies*, tr. S. Gilbert in Sartre; *Altona, Men Without Shadows, The Flies*, Penguin Books, Harmondsworth, 1962.
———.(1944) *In Camera* (*Huis Clos*), tr. S. Gilbert in E.M. Browne (ed.) *Three European Plays*, Penguin Books, Harmondsworth, 1958.
———.(1944) "Paris Alive: The Republic of Silence", tr. L. Kirstein, *Atlantic Monthly*, CLXXIV, Dec.
———.(1945) *The Age of Reason*, tr. E. Sutton, Penguin Books, Harmondsworth, 1961.
———.(1945) "American Cities" in his *Literary and Philosophical Essays*, tr. A Michelson, Hutchinson, London, 1955.
———.(1945) "The Case for Responsible Literature", tr. N. Galitzine, *Partisan Review*, XII, 3, Summer.
———.(1945) "Individualism and Conformism in the United States" in *Literary and Philosophical Essays*.
———.(1945) *The Reprieve*, tr. E. Sutton, Penguin Books, Harmondsworth, 1963.
———.(1946) "American Novelists in French Eyes", *Atlantic Monthly*, CLXXVIII, August.
———.(1946) *The Chips are Down* (*Les Jeux sont faits*) tr. L. Varese, Rider, London, 1951.
———.(1946) *Existentialism and Humanism*, tr. P. Mairet, Methuen, London, 1948.
———.(1946) "Forgers of Myths: The Young Playwrights of France", *Theatre Arts*, XXX, June.
———.(1946) Letter in *New York Herald Tribune* (European Edition), Nov. 20.

———.(1946) "Materialism and Revolution" in *Literary and Philosophical Essays*.

———.(1946) *Men Without Shadows (Morts sans sépulture)*, tr. K. Black in *Altona, Men Without Shadows, The Flies*.

———.(1946) "New York, the Colonial City" in *Literary and Philosophical Essays*.

———.(1946) *Portrait of the Anti-Semite*, tr. E. de Maung, Secker and Warburg, London, 1948.

———.(1946) *The Respectful Prostitute*, tr. K. Black, in Sartre; *Two Plays*, Penguin Books, Harmondsworth, 1965.

———.(1946) "We Write for Our Time", *Meanjin*, VI, Summer 1947.

———.(1947) "Americans and their Myths", *Nation*, CLXV, October.

———.(1947) *Baudelairs*, tr. M. Turnell, Hamish Hamilton, London, 1949.

———.(1947) "I Discovered Jazz in America", *Saturday Review of Literature*, XXX, Nov.

———.(1947) Lettre-Préface to F. Jeanson; *Le Probleme moral et la pensee de Sartre*, Editions du Myrte, Paris.

———.(1947) "The Responsibility of the Writer", tr. B. Askwith in *Reflections on Our Age*, Allan Wingate, London, 1948.

———.(1947) *What is Literature?*, tr. B. Frechtman, Methuen, London, 1967.

———.(1947) "The Word as Mirror", *Saturday Review of Literature*, XXX, Dec. 6.

———.(1948) *Crime Passionnel (Les Mains Sales)*, tr. K. Black, Methuen, London, 1961.

———.(1948) *In the Mesh (L'Engrenage)*, tr. M. Savill, Dakers, London, 1954.

———.(1948) "Nathalie Sarraute" in his *Situations*, tr. B. Eisler, Hamish Hamilton, London, 1965.

———.(1949) "Drôle d'amitié", *Les Temps Modernes*, 49, Nov.

———.(1949) *Iron in the Soul (La Mort dans L'âme)* tr. G. Hopkins, Penguin Books, Harmondsworth, 1963.

———.*et al* (1949) *Entretiens sur la politique*, Gallimard, Paris.

———.(1951) *The Devil and the Good Lord*, tr. K. Black, Vintage Books, New York, 1960.

———.(1951) "The Living Gide" in *Situations*.

———.(1952) "Reply to Albert Camus" in *Situations*.

———.(1952) *Saint Genet: Actor and Martyr*, tr. B. Frechtman, W.H. Allen, London, 1964.

———.(1952, 1954) *The Communists and Peace*, tr. I. Clephane, Hamish Hamilton, London, 1969.

———.(1953) Interview, *Libération*, Nov. 4.

———.(1954) *Kean*, tr. K. Black in Sartre: *Three Plays*, Penguin Books, Harmondsworth, 1969.

———.(1955) "... Said Jean-Paul Sartre", (Interview) tr. R. Drell, *Yale French Studies*, 16, Winter 1955-56.

———.(1956-57) *The Spectre of Stalin*, tr. I. Clephane, Hamish Hamilton, London, 1969.

———.(1957) "Interview with Oliver Todd", *Listener*, LVII, June 6.
———.(1958) "Of Rats and Men", in *Situations*.
———.(1958) "La Réponse d'Henri Alleg", *Les Temps Modernes*, 145, Jan.-Feb.
———.(1958) "A Victory", tr. J. Calder, Preface to Henri Alleg; *The Question*, John Calder, London, 1958.
———.(1960) *Altona (Les Séquestrés d'Altona)* tr. S. and G. Lesson in Sartre; *Altona, Men Without Shadows, The Flies*.
———.(1960) *Critique de la raison dialectique*, Gallimard, Paris.
———.(1960) *Sartre on Cuba* (no tr.), Ballantine Books, New York, 1961.
———.(1960) *Search for a Method (Question de methode)*, tr. H. E. Barnes, Vintage Books, New York, 1968.
———.(1960) "To Show, To Demonstrate" (Interview), Yale French Studies, 30.
———.(1961) "An Interview with Jean-Paul Sartre" (O.F. Pucciani), *The Tulane Drama Review*, V, 3.
———.(1961) "Merleau-Ponty" in *Situations*.
———.(1961) Preface to F. Fanon; *The Wretched of the Earth*, tr. C. Farrington, Penguin Books, Harmondsworth, 1967.
———.(1961) "Sartre talks to Tynan—I and II" (Interview), *Observer*, London, June 18, 25.
———.(1963) Foreword to Laing and Cooper, op. cit.
———.(1963) *Words* tr. I. Clephane, Penguin Books, Harmondsworth, 1967.
———.(1964) "A Long Bitter-Sweet Madness" (Interview), tr. A. Hartley, *Encounter*, XXII, June.
———.(1964) "Sartre on the Nobel Prize", tr. R. Howard, *New York Review of Books*, I, Dec. 17.
———.(1964) "L'Universel singulier" in *Kierkegaard vivant*, Gallimard, coll. "Idees", Paris, 1966.
———.(1965) "Jean-Paul Sartre", *Playboy Interviews* Playboy Press, Chicago, 1967.
———.(1965) "Why I Will not Go to the United States", *Nation*, CC, 16, April 19. See also a cable from Sartre cited in "Up All Night", *Nation*, CC, 22, May 31, 1965.
———.(1969) "Itinerary of a Thought" (Interview), *New Left Review*, 58, Nov.-Dec.
———.(1971) *Gustave Flaubert de 1821 a 1857*, I, II, (III, 1972).
———.(1973) "On Maoism: An Interview with Jean-Paul Sartre", tr. R. D'Amico, *Telos*, 16, Summer.
———.(1975) Interview with Michel Contat, *Le Nouvel Observateur*, 554, 555, 556.
Schafer, R. "The Psychoanalytic Vision of Reality", *International Journal of Psychoanalysis*, 51, 1970.
Schmidt, A. *The Concept of Nature in Marx*, New Left Books, London, 1971.
Searles, H. "The Effort to Drive the Other Person Crazy", *British Journal of Medical Psychology*, XXXII, pt. I, 1959.

Sedgwick, P. "Peter Sedgwick Meditates on the Acceptability of R.D. Laing", *Listener* 2251, 18 May 1972.

———."Self, Symptom and Society" in R. Boyers and R. Orrill (eds.); *Laing and Anti-Psychiatry*, Penguin Books, Harmondsworth, 1972. (Originally ibid., *Salmagundi*, 16, Spring 1971.)

Solomon, R. *From Rationalism to Existentialism: The Existentialists and their Nineteenth Century Background*, Harper and Row, New York, 1972.

Stern, K. *The Flight from Woman*, Allen and Unwin, London, 1966.

Storr, A. *The Dynamics of Creation*, Secker and Warburg, London, 1972.

———.*Human Destructiveness* Chatto-Heinemann, London, 1972.

Szasz, T. *The Myth of Mental Illness*, Delta, New York, 1961.

Thody, P. *Sartre: A Biographical Introduction*, Studio Vista, London, 1971.

Trilling, L. *Sincerity and Authenticity*, Harvard University Press, Cambridge, Mass., 1972.

Wahl, J. *Philosophies of Existence*, Routledge and Kegan Paul, London, 1969.

Weber, M. "Politics as a Vocation" in Gerth and Mills, op. cit.

———.*The Protestant Ethic and the Rise of Capitalism*, Allen and Unwin, London, 1930.

———."Science as a Vocation", in Gerth and Mills, op. cit.

Winnicott, D.W. *Collected Papers*, Tavistock, London, 1958.

———. *The Maturational Processes and the Facilitating Environment: Studies in the Theory of Emotional Development*, Hogarth Press, London, 1965.

———. *Playing and Reality*, Tavistock, London, 1971.

# Index